Healthy Heart and Mind:
It's ALL a Practice

SHANNA HAUN

Student Stories
Collected by Jan Sokoloff Harness

DEDICATION

To my family of origin, my family of creation and all my amazing students who propel me forward.

DISCLAIMER

Table of Contents

ACKNOWLEDGMENTS

It takes a village to raise a child and it definitely takes a community of people to write and publish a book! Thank you to my cheerleader and editor, Jan Sokoloff Harness, for inspiring this entire project and giving me guidance and encouragement along the way. To my wonderful husband, Matt, for taking all the photos, designing the book cover, doing all things technical and never losing his patience with me! I am truly blessed. To my children, Mackenzie and Aaron, my mother, Sylvie Radvinsky, and my sister, Tami Pratt, for their support, enthusiasm and unwavering belief in the outcome of this book.

To my first official reader and back cover contributor, Maureen O'Brien Salz! You gave me courage and I am eternally grateful. To my circuit ladies and Blue Valley Rec students – you make my already fun job even more fabulous. Your questions, interest and enthusiasm are a constant source of inspiration and motivation! To Molly Keehn and the entire staff of the Blue Valley Rec Center for providing a wonderful place to work and creating a space where fitness is so accessible. To Anne Sullivan, all my peeps at Lululemon® Leawood and the entire Lululemon company for reinforcing big goal setting and embracing imperfection! To my early readers: Lezlie Revelle Zucker, Yara Nielsenshultz, Laura Intfen, Anne Schultz, Barbara Cason and Jamie Thompson. Your input was invaluable!

Finally, thank you to my father, Israel Radvinsky. I wish you were physically present to witness this project. I miss you and your amazing hugs. I am so grateful that you were my dad. So much of this book is inspired by all that you taught me. I love you.

I. LIVING LIFE ... AS A "PRACTICER"

Since it is my career and passion, the topic of "living healthy" frequently comes up in discussions. Regardless of a woman's age, size or life experience, whether she is my student or we just happen to meet, I encounter the same themes and typically self-berating tones: "My balance sucks. Will I ever improve?" "I used to be so flexible. Will I ever be able to touch my toes again?" "I have a bad (fill in the blank)." "You wouldn't know from looking at me, but I've been exercising for years."

The fact that I repeatedly hear the same questions and comments speaks to my heart. I want a revolution of us women thinking and speaking differently, positively and compassionately about our bodies. Let's **recognize** and give ourselves credit for our strengths. Let's positively shift the paradigm of what we "absolutely know" about ourselves. Let's put an end to silent comparisons with other women. Let's believe wholeheartedly that no matter what other women look like, no matter their abilities – perfection does not exist and is not the goal.

Perfect does not exist. Practice is highly achievable! Let's change the way we ask questions to be empowered and knowledge seeking: "How do I improve my balance, flexibility and strength?" "How can I measure improvement?" "What are things I can do to feel stronger and have more energy?" These types of questions set us up for success right from the start.

Healthy Heart and Mind: It's ALL a Practice is my personal journey to living a healthy life on all levels – mind, body and soul. It is my approach to living life as a "practicer" traveling among fellow "practicers."

Within these pages, I share stories of my family of origin and how it shaped my view of the world. I share stories of my family of creation that motivate my choices every day. I share a philosophy of empowerment. Yes, ideas and potential strategies that I find beneficial are included. However, I firmly believe that you have the right to create your own definition of what living healthy means for you. You get to decide how to go about it all **and** you are allowed to change your definition along the way. Life changes and priorities evolve. I tell all my students that while in class, I am a guide, but they know themselves best and always have the right to veto anything I say. When need be, they do and it is a beautiful sight!

My amazing students are a variety of ages, sizes, backgrounds … and they are all inspiring definitions of living healthy. The majority of them are women, whether I'm teaching yoga, Pilates or strength training. More than half are between the ages of 50 and 75. Yet, I don't teach special "50-plus" classes. I teach all-level classes. And, I tell you now: 50, 60, 70 years old does not look the same as it did when I was a kid! And it is not just because I have reached 40! Every day, I am inspired by their fabulousness and couldn't pass up the opportunity to share some of their stories with you.

Healthy Heart and Mind: It's ALL a Practice gives us a way to redirect the tone in typical discussions about our health and fitness level. Let's make "No Judgment!" and "No Comparisons Allowed!" the norm. Better yet, let's create a space where those reminders are not even necessary!

Healthy longevity – those two words are my mantra … my hope. How we move in our body, our living posture, speaks volumes regarding the quality of our daily life. When I look around, I always notice how people move. Everywhere I go, I observe issues in the hips, lower back and neck. I see favoring of one side over another. I wonder if those characteristics cause pain or suffering. I wonder at the possibility of eliminating or reducing existing pain and/or suffering. Would enhanced body awareness make a positive difference? Evidence from all my years of teaching offers a resounding, "YES! Most definitely!" It's never, ever too late to improve the quality of one's life on all levels – physically, mentally and emotionally.

I feel driven to teach body awareness and ways to use that awareness to move and live well. Time and time again, I have witnessed the dramatic impact to my students' lives. Just because we are getting older does not mean we have to resign ourselves to ever-growing aches and pains. I cannot and will not promise a cure. I **can** share a management style that has proven helpful for many and an approach, a mindset, that can assist the process.

I love seeing my students transform to standing taller and feeling stronger. They say they hear my voice in their head as they move about their days: send your shoulders back, lengthen your spine, root down in your feet, on and on. It's fantastic!

In turn, my students inspire me. Those who are older than I am are examples of everything I hope and want for myself as each decade approaches. They have vigor, power and joy. They make living longer look mah'velous!

Taking the journey individually … and together

On our road to healthy longevity, there is no perfect. There is no judgment. It is all a practice. We are never done until the big "D." The journey and the learning are forever – as we know forever to be.

I think the journey, the learning, the living, are all exciting. In becoming more aware, we travel inward and discover new aspects of ourselves. With that awareness, we are more empowered in all areas of our life. We have a positive impact on those around us.

With every day and every decade, we get to define what matters most to us right now. We get to change our definition with time and experience. We get to choose how we see ourselves.

On my journey, I choose to see myself not as a size or a weight. I choose to see myself as a teacher, sharing a positive, empowered, and compassionate message of what living healthy can mean. Let's feel good in our own skin. Let's inspire others to do the same!

Class Descriptions

To give you an idea of the classes mentioned throughout this book:

Hatha Yoga (60 minutes): The way I interpret Hatha Yoga is to teach one pose at a time and provide options for varying degrees of intensity. We deliberately set up each pose and consciously explore how our physical alignment affects our endurance, strength, breath and state of mind. This is not a "flow-style" class. We may never do a tricep push-up (Chaturanga Dandasana). I do not use Downward-Facing Dog (Adho Mukha Svanasana) as a transition pose. Yet, it never ceases to impress the students how challenged they can feel by holding a properly aligned pose! The goals of the practice are to reduce tension, increase flexibility, improve balance and feel good. My hope is that students leave feeling taller and less stressed! The class is appropriate for all fitness levels.

Small Group Women-Only Circuit (60 minutes): This is a shared personal training session (limited to seven women). My mission is to help women feel strong, empowered and inspired by building strength intelligently and safely. The class design is a short group warm-up followed by approximately 20 minutes of group strength training for the calves, thighs, glutes and arms. We then do two rounds of seven 1-minute stations. Each station has an individual focus: cardio, balance, plank, abs, arms, chest/back and legs. We always end the class with stretching (typically with a foam roller).

This is not a "boot camp" and there is no shouting. I pay very close attention to everyone's physical alignment. Students always have the right to veto any exercise and we come up with modifications to make any exercise more appropriate. This is a supportive, positive and non-competitive environment.

Mat Pilates (30 minutes): I try to remove the intimidation of a Pilates practice while still keeping the focus on precision and alignment. We concentrate on the fundamentals while exploring options within each exercise for varying degrees of intensity. A Pilates practice tones, strengthens and builds long, lean muscles and a stronger, leaner core. The class is 30 minutes so that students can attend both Pilates and yoga, back-to-back, without feeling overly fatigued. Many students have found the benefits of their Pilates practice to strengthen their yoga practice. Others are grateful to have a 30-minute option for exercising as their lives are extremely busy.

II. ROOTS

My dad loved his audio tape recorder. He also loved surprising, teasing and catching us off guard. During many family discussions, he would pull out the tape recorder and reveal that it had been recording us for the past 20 minutes. Sometimes, we would see that it was in the room with us. When questioned, Dad would lie and say the red light just meant the power was plugged in but nothing was recording.

Eventually, he had to prove it to us. But, with all his machinations, we have quite a collection of uninhibited conversations and they are incredible.

Decades later, I am so grateful to hear all of us as we were in real time – no pretense, unaware of putting on a show. My grandparents would speak in their blend of Russian, Hebrew and English – depending on what they wanted us to understand and what was first available in their minds.

My younger sister and I would argue with all the ugliness that we could. My mom would get irritated with my dad and warn us to stop with our roughhousing or someone was going to end up hurt

– and she was always right. The majority of the tapes are filled with laughter; the kind with side aches and tears. Those tapes exhibit our truth in the moment; they are a magical and invaluable family record.

Shortly after my father passed away, I pulled out those dusty tapes. On one of them, I was 13 years old and my dad was asking me what I wanted to do when I grew up. In my sing-songy way, I said, "I don't know." After a pause I added, "I know I want to be healthy." Hearing this conversation as an adult felt surreal. I completely forgot I ever said or even thought that as a kid. Why on earth would that have occurred to me?

My 13-year-old Self

At 13, I was at the end of my fascination with serious ballet classes and they had become too expensive for my parents to afford. I was not good at any team sports; I was always one of the last kids selected during PE or recess games. I felt inept at all things physical other than dancing and that didn't seem to do me any good – even or especially at school dances.

I felt outside the group. I was awkward and geeky but never felt as smart as others presumed. "Coolness" was highly valued and totally elusive. The only place I felt I really fit in was with my family. So I clung to the fact that no matter what my peers thought, my family thought the world of me. I did well enough but I wasn't passionate about whatever I was doing. I felt kind of odd and aimless.

Living Sick

Shortly after that recording, my father's father died. Deda (Russian for *grandfather*) wanted to see me become a Bat Mitzvah and then passed away a few months later. He was sick for many years and died of a heart attack at the age of 74. His was the first "real" death my family experienced.

After open-heart surgery eight years prior, Deda's life had become a blend of lethargy, eating foods he didn't like and arguing with my Baba (Russian for *grandmother*) about what she had prepared for him. She hid the saltshaker from him, yelled at him about his demands for a hamburger and then cried and kissed his bald head.

After Deda died, Baba's life purpose also died. She spent the next nine years focused on feeling sick and getting sicker. She frequently complained of feeling sick or alluding to her potential, imminent death – in stereotypical, guilt-inducing comments.

As a teen and in my early 20s, I found myself watching my grandmother with a see-sawing blend of silent criticism, overwhelming frustration, resentment for the kind of attention she craved, fear of her death, lack of empathy, concern for her mental, emotional and physical states, grief for her previous vibrancy and all the while – love.

How could a person be sick for so many years without it being treatable or identifiable? And, if she was so worried, why would she continue to make the same choices about her diet and habits? Baba went from doctor to doctor accumulating prescriptions, conflicting information and getting all worked up.

It drove my father crazy until he checked out of the situation entirely and told my mother to "just deal with it." Ultimately, my grandmother's body began to shut down. I think a part of her felt vindicated that she was finally dying of diseases that had names – lung cancer, kidney failure …

On my mother's side, Zady (Yiddish for *grandfather*) died a painful death of liver failure at 75. In his final weeks, he held nothing down and withered away. It was awful and helpless to witness. Thankfully sans suffering, my Bubbe (Yiddish for *grandmother*) died quietly in her sleep at the age of 77. All the grandparents died in their 70s. I now know it is way too young but, at the time, it seemed expected and unsurprising to all of us.

Dying Before Age 70

Based on family history, I (and I think everyone) thought Dad would live into his 70s. At the same time, in the year prior to his passing, I shared fears with my husband that Dad's health seemed to be declining. His decades-long habit of smoking, eating large portions rapidly and being an erratic exerciser appeared to be taking its toll. He started feeling ill and got sick from eating any amount of food. He became out of breath from the smallest activity. Hindsight being 20/20, these are textbook symptoms for risk of heart attack. Dad visited the doctor once but fearing what the doctor might say, he lied about his symptoms.

November 26, 2007, Dad was sitting in his chair at the end of a Monday workday, on the phone with my sister discussing the most recent University of Kansas football game, when the call dropped. My sister tried to call back but he wouldn't pick up, so she called to see if I was on the phone with him. Our mom was with me and we were getting ready to leave for my yoga class. I thought my sister was needlessly worried and was about to dismiss her concern until she stated that she was at their house.

Startled at her quick alarm, I heard her walk into the house and say, "Dad? Dad? Dad! Oh my God, Shanna, get over here right now!" and she hung up on me. I later learned that as Mom and I were rushing to the house, my sister had to drag our father out of his recliner and onto the floor, apply CPR, all while staying on the phone with the 911 dispatcher.

When my mom and I arrived at the house, my first concern was for my sister. I just wanted to hold her and calm her because I knew she was traumatized. I was sure that Dad was fine. All I could think about as the paramedics were working on him, the neighbors were standing outside and the lights of the fire trucks were glaring, was that Dad was going to be pissed as hell at the commotion we had caused. And then, he never woke up.

I had spoken to him several times that day – as was typical for us. How could he be gone and how was I going to tell my kids? How was I going to live life without my Dad? It wasn't supposed to happen for at least 10 more years, he was only 59. I am a planner and based on our family history, I was supposed to have more time with him.

Now, as I write this, it is five years since his death. There is a richness and beauty to pain. There is a humbling to living life with a gap in your heart and understanding that it will always be there. That the gap is certain to grow bigger with each loved one that you outlive. I have an appreciation for my past and am grateful for the plethora of memories and experiences that motivate me today.

I miss my Dad so much. I was a superstar in his eyes. I want to live well – for myself, for him, for my family of origin, for the family I created and for all my students. At 13, all I knew was that

I wanted to be healthy when I grew up. Today, striving to live well pushes me forward and gives purpose to my life. Living well feeds my soul.

III. EAT, EAT!!

As a kid, I saw how the family's relationship with food was out of balance. Today, I see how it affected the overall quality of our lives. Energy level, mood and desire (or lack thereof) to do anything were all impacted. As a family, we would go in waves of high activity to being lazy around the house.

Baba frequently chastised me for the personal affront of not eating whatever she had worked so hard to prepare. When visiting, her first question was always, "Are you hungry?" After years of that question one would think that I would plan better, but most often I wasn't hungry and replied, "No." In a thick Russian accent she would say, "Okay, I make you fruit." My reply, "But, Baba, I am not hungry." She would balk as though I uttered nonsense, "You don't need to be hungry for fruit!" or, "You mean you are not even going to try it? How hungry do you have to be to try this?!!"

I was always incredulous. For me, visiting was solely about spending time with her. Unless I was hungry, I didn't want to be bothered with the distraction of food. For me, get-togethers are all about the people I am with. Food is very secondary, almost an afterthought of, "Oh yeah, people like to eat, will expect and look forward to it. Munching is sort of satisfying." I never figured out or was too stubborn to lie and just say *yes*, simply to make her happy.

For Baba, food was love. She was an excellent cook but it was all loaded. Every summer, she would make delicious strawberry dumplings (we called them *kreplach*) that we then topped with full-fat sour cream and strawberry "preserves," which was at least one cup of sugar, mixed with some strawberries and water heated on the stove.

Everything was like that; full fat, full grease, full, full, full ... but, never enough ...

Opposite Extremes

At home, my mother went on health kicks. Ironically, it is similar to how I eat today. But at the time, all I could think was, "What the hell is wheat germ?" I just wanted sweet cereals and with everything else I added ketchup; pasta, eggs, chicken, beef, especially vegetables. Ketchup was a food group unto itself and made everything taste yummier.

Mom was always experimenting and trying new things, new brands, new recipes and the rest of us constantly resisted. Today, I feel bad for the pains in the asses that we were to her, but that is how we were – much of the time. Every once in a while, Mom would hit a homerun, like when we "discovered" artichokes. Of course, we dipped every single leaf into rich mayonnaise with lemon juice! Yum! Oy.

I never thought about food unless I was hungry, but everyone around me loved to talk about it. Whatever meal we were eating, often the topic of what to eat next was discussed. To this day, I can't really think about food unless I am hungry. Thinking about it makes me feel unpleasantly full – as though describing it means I am eating it – and there is no room in my belly.

Guaranteed Health??!

Around my teen years, anxiety kicked in and I started to develop a fear of eating and sickness. I hated the idea of being sick, especially the kind that would cause me to throw up. So, I started researching. Were there any "safe" foods that would not cause illness? Were there any strategies that could guarantee my health? There was no Internet so I was trying to research by observing behaviors and comments of those around me without admitting my fears.

Obviously, there is no such thing as life sans illness but looking back is a fascinating and heart-aching exercise. Trying to keep the details of my fear a secret from my family – because I knew I sounded ridiculous – was also trying and tiring.

Eventually, my secret came out. There was more compassion and love than judgment. They didn't necessarily get it but they all had junk of their own that they were managing. I didn't have to be perfect for them to love and accept me.

In sharing my secret with them, I still felt anxious, but far less vulnerable and paranoid. They could tease me in a loving way; threaten to make me eat octopus or meat that was left out all night. And, I could laugh at myself and with them.

Adulthood Does Not Mean Perfection

I'd love to say that I'm no longer afraid of illness or throwing up but that would be an outrageous lie. Illness still makes me edgy, throwing up freaks me out and inspires me to negotiate with any higher being.

Before my husband and I ever had children, he promised me that kid's vomit would be his domain – and it mostly has been. It turns out that my response to them throwing up is like his response to their crying for no obvious reason: he freezes and I feel completely equipped.

When the kids were little and got sick, I felt the need to apologize to them for my shortcomings. I felt so guilty but also paralyzed with fear. In addition, I was afraid that my fears would become their fears and I couldn't bear to pass on that burden. So, I explained that my fears were completely irrational, no logic or truth to them.

The kids looked at me with reassurance that they loved having Dad by their side in sickness. He was comforting. I am good at other things. Simple as that. Aren't kids wonderful?

Once, my dad told me, "You know, Shanna, you would be perfect if you didn't have this fear." First of all, I love the fact that he was that delusional. Over time, I have also come to realize that my fear and anxiety, as irrational as they are, make me empathetic.

I understand fear. I understand struggle – no matter the subject. Fear and struggle are part of the human experience. Not one of us is immune. We all just have our own unique combination! The question is, how much power do we give over to fear … or to whatever we struggle with? How much do we let it restrict our lives or drain our energy? Some time ago, I made my decision and I strive to live by that decision each day.

Fear Doesn't Get a Vote

Fear cannot rule my motivations or drive. It does not get a deciding vote in any situation. I can acknowledge fear's points, its effects on my psyche and emotions. However, avoiding fear cannot be the exclusive reason I say "yes" or "no" to any question.

If fear rules, then I am enslaved. And – I've enslaved myself. I refuse to let that be my reality. Fear and anxiety can have a voice but not **THE** voice. They cannot win. I must win. Every freakin' day! It's not always pretty. Some days the struggle feels bigger than others but the theme remains: fear does not get the deciding vote.

We are not our struggles. In any moment, we are how we manage our struggles. **We are all that we accomplish in spite of our struggles.** So, take a deep breath and know that you are not alone. Our struggles aren't always visible to one another but we all share in the fact that we've got them. You are good. You are doing the best you can in this moment. Let me repeat, YOU ARE DOING THE BEST YOU CAN IN THIS MOMENT. And so is that other woman who doesn't appear to have the exact same struggles as you. Guess what? She is desperately struggling with something that you have either mastered or would never even identify as a problem. And she thinks **YOU** are amazing and strong and brave.

We are all that we accomplish in spite of our struggles
Please choose to see your many, many accomplishments

A Note About the Student Stories

Jan Sokoloff Harness conducted interviews with the women selected for this book. She was curious about how the women perceived their weight. Did they weigh themselves? Did they care about the number? Each woman's response was different. Some said their number flat out, some said their typical weight range, other said they either didn't know, didn't care or that it was less than when they began their fitness journey!

We decided that including the specific answers in the individual stories was antithetical to the messages within this book. What was truly interesting were the variety in responses. A woman is more than her weight. Her definition of feeling and living healthy is not dependent upon a number on the scale. A successful health story is not about pounds lost but **life gained**. We think all of the student stories personify a transformation to living a healthier life on all levels; mind, body and soul.

MAHSHID HESANI

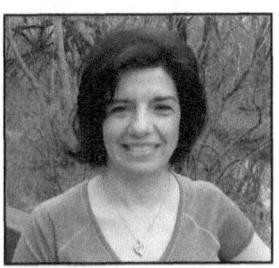

50 years old

In the midst of a divorce, two daughters

Ask Mahshid Hesani a question about yoga or Pilates, and her answers, her laughter and her infectious joy immediately surround you. She speaks in exclamation points, eager to share the differences she sees in herself – and just as eager to encourage others to try yoga, Pilates, whatever speaks to their soul. A teacher, Mahshid says the lessons she has learned during her first year of regular exercise help her feel whole, connecting mind, body and spirit.

I look at myself in the mirror and I'm happy. I can see the strength in me.

I came here from Iran 30 years ago and I was not into exercise; I never did it before. Well, I tried different things, but I was too lazy! And it always felt forced, not natural. But, about a year ago, I was in the middle of a divorce, and my brothers said, "Mahshid, you have to do yoga." So I asked my friends at work about yoga, and one of them said it was very good. I thought, "I will try one time and see if I like it."

That first time in Shanna's yoga class, it was hard. I was shaking. Yoga has a language of its own; it's like a different foreign language to me. When Shanna talked about being grounded, energy coming from the outside, it was all a new language. But it was peaceful, and I thought, "I could do this and be a good role model for my kids."

My two girls, they don't exercise. I can't tell them, "You have to do it," if I don't do it. They need to see me do it. Now, little by little, they are taking baby steps. I showed the youngest one last week, one pose. Next, I will show her another pose. Baby steps. Just like yoga! When I did the plank first, I couldn't do it for one second! Now I can stay in it. I show my friends, I say, "Come see my plank!"

I do yoga almost every day and I talk about it all the time. My friends, they probably get tired of me talking about it! But let me tell you, I was on sleeping pills before yoga and I didn't want to be. Now, I sleep better and better and I don't need a pill. My mental health is much more open, you know what I mean? Like it was foggy before and now it's not. Everything is more clear for me.

You ask how much I weigh. I don't know. I haven't weighed. That's not my thing. People get so obsessed with weight. They just look at the numbers. Why? Do you have energy? Do you have muscles? Do you have strength? Why say, "If today I weigh 130, I'm fine. If today I weigh 131, oh no!" That's not accurate. That's no way to measure.

I look at the inner me and I can see the strength in me. I walk like this, shoulders back and I feel the inner strength. I didn't have this before, even when I was younger. And I think, "Where did that come from?" It comes from yoga and a good teacher. A good teacher makes all the difference. One hour of yoga with Shanna is better than any medicine. It's medicine for your soul. It clears your mind and how you look at life. Why pay for insurance and medicine and not pay for Shanna? She helps mentally, physically – and you look better!

Every time I look at myself in the mirror and I'm happy, that's it. That's good. I'm happy externally and internally – and other people see it too. The PE teacher at the school where I teach asked me, "Did you do surgery? There's something about you changed. You're glowing and I can see the energy surrounding you." That's what I feel too. And I say, "No surgery! Yoga!"

For me, yoga is a question of priority, priority, priority. I refuse to compromise yoga. That's my one hour for me; that's my priority.

Going through a divorce, moving to a different country, I've gone through a lot. But since I started with Shanna, I can see her mind; I can hear her say, "Connect your mind, body and spirit," and I know it's up to us to do that. It's up to us to come to class. It doesn't matter which part of the world you are from or what your culture is. Body is body. Mental health is mental health. Doing yoga doesn't start or stop with any culture.

I enjoy this. I enjoy yoga. And I enjoy life.

IV. EMPOWERED CHOICE

Practicing yoga, exercising in general, and eating a balanced and healthy diet are tools that help me **manage** my life. If I don't exercise, I feel tired and bee-yotchy – as my daughter and I like to say because no one in the house is allowed to say that I am being the real thing even if it is true! So, I'd rather work out and feel "good tired" than be stagnant and feel "pissed tired."

Sugar dramatically affects my mood, increases my anxiety and overall makes me feel awful. I have to go through withdrawal to clear its effects from my system. Therefore, I choose to avoid it – at least most of the time!

Depriving myself only increases my cravings, so I eat healthy foods that leave me feeling good. I also have dark chocolate covered almonds and popcorn most days because they also make me feel good. I eat what I love and I love what I eat. I eat for energy and overall wellbeing.

I've had a smoothie for breakfast and salad for lunch every day for over 10 years and I still love and look forward to them both. I might eat eggs at some point in the afternoon then a healthy dinner my wonderful husband prepares or a second salad.

Sometimes, a late evening snack if I get hungry because I don't want hunger to interrupt my sleep.

Ingredients adjust with the seasons and news of what may be beneficial. Check the "Resources" chapter for my specific, ever-changing recipes. Fifteen years ago, I would not have imagined that I would be consuming hemp and chia seeds on a daily basis. Ch'ch'ch' chia was a toy of some sort.

Positive, Mindful Routines

I am a routine eater and comforted by not thinking too much about what to eat at the next meal. I enjoy spending my mental and physical energies in other ways. Cooking for my family every evening would be agonizing and energy draining. No one needs that kind of vibe in the house (especially from the mom).

For many years, I struggled with guilt over the fact that I really don't like to cook. **But, guilt did not motivate me to do anything differently!** So, I decided to shift my focus to one of gratitude. I am grateful that both kids prepare foods they want to eat and have for a very long time. I am tremendously grateful to be married to a man who enjoys cooking for the two of us AND works with all of my dietary preferences without resentment.

I work best and feel most successful with positive, mindful routines in my life. I can and I do adapt as life changes. I also frequently reassess: is my current routine still positively serving my life or does anything need tweaking? Is there a mood of discontent or unnecessary stress surrounding anything? I don't (or at least I try not to) ignore the subtle messages from life.

When grappling with any decision, I visualize my foreseeable options and see each one through to its potential result. I make what feels like the best decision in the moment and then evaluate results based on evidence.

This strategy pertains to the mundane as well as the significant decisions: what I eat, how I spend my time and energy, what I purchase, what I wear, etc. I strive to make all my decisions with full awareness and empowered choice.

Avoiding My Inner Victim/Martyr

My nature easily goes to victimhood-martyrdom or bad temper. I find those aspects of myself ugly and embarrassing. I minimize their potential by being and holding myself accountable to be fully aware.

I won't make decisions relying solely on someone else's influence – even if they are experts. Experts are providing knowledge based on their experience up to the moment the advice is given. As they learn more in their given field, they adjust what they advise.

I know this to be true for myself as a teacher. What I teach in my classes today has dramatically evolved over the years. Sometimes, I wish I could go back to my early students and apologize!! Therefore, I listen and consider others' perspectives, contemplate my options and make the best decision I can for myself.

Whatever decision I make, I do not hold an expert or anyone else accountable. This way, I own it completely. Whether I am right or wrong, I can live with it. If I mess up, I can reflect and strive to minimize whatever pattern led to that misstep.

I am the navigator of my life. I make and live with my choices. No one is going to do that for me. Since I have to live with them, I am highly motivated to make the best ones for me. I have learned to trust myself most no matter what, because my intentions for myself are good. I've got my back.

Ultimately, you've got your back. You are living with you. Deep down inside, you know best what makes you feel empowered, happy and strong. I hope this book proves helpful, informative and inspires positive change in your life – however **YOU** define it.

I always let my students know that they have the power to veto any instruction I give. As long as they are being safe, I will not interfere. No matter what, you have to be able to count on yourself. You have to be able to trust yourself most!

Mind Your Inner Voice

Trust your inner intelligence … that trustworthy voice deep within. Try to heed it when the messages are subtle and quiet. Avoiding or rejecting inner messages at the outset can cause them to grow louder. Louder messages typically mean imminent drama or injury. If ignored for too long, the messages can also go mute – an even worse scenario.

Physically, pain is inner communication. There's some garbled noise in the joint. What is the point of powering through? How exactly would that prove beneficial? Powering through always comes at a cost. Is it worth it?

Is powering through worth the time, effort and process of recovery? Unless we are professional athletes who've signed up for the risk or are working through a prior injury with a professional, it is hard to come up with a justifiable reason to move through pain.

I believe powering through is the same as ignoring. It is potentially being rude to yourself. Instead, stop, reset, then mindfully decide whether it makes sense to continue and to what intensity. What is intelligent in this moment?

We receive inner messages all the time. They come from our body, our emotions, our thoughts and we respond accordingly. Those internal messages are typically gifts, forewarnings, and may not easily return. How often do we pay attention? How often do we give those messages a voice? How often do we ignore them? Would we ever ignore someone else's voice in the same way?

If our pattern is to constantly tell our inner voice to shut up, then eventually it will … until we have a major problem. Mind your inner voice. Trust your inner voice. The more you tune in to it, the more it will serve you positively. The more you tune in to it, the more efficiently you will hear it.

While teaching, I'm often questioned about the difference between pain and discomfort. We are seeking our edge. We are looking for sensory input and trying to navigate our journey safely. Sensations can be confusing. I explain pain as sharp and shooting. It has a very specific location and can be easily identified. Pain is especially alarming when felt in a joint and should not be ignored. I always advise releasing a painful position slowly and carefully.

Discomfort is broad. It's unspecific. Students usually show me the source of their discomfort by waving a hand over an area; typically it is around whatever muscle we are focusing on. For discomfort, I give them a thumbs up! The students get to determine intensity but mild discomfort is part of the process of change. Understanding the difference between pain and appropriate discomfort is an ongoing exercise in discernment and improves with time and practice.

Inner Wisdom vs. Inner Fear

Let's honor the voice within – not the fear within – but the wisdom within. The two sound totally different. Inner wisdom comes from our core, our gut, our essence. Inner wisdom is quiet, it's clear and may only be a phrase. It's our inner truth with a capital "T."

Fear, anxiety and self-doubt come from the brain. Their messages often conflict, feel scattered and haywire. They are usually given too much attention! I call the anxious, fearful thoughts "monkey mind." Anxiety and fear are fast thoughts, all jumbled and bouncing around – like monkeys in a cage. The more attention we give, responding to them on that level, the louder and more rambunctious they become. They might be true'ish statements but they are situational and any "guidance" gleaned will not serve us positively on a consistent basis.

Let's make room for the voice that serves us best. Intuition, inner wisdom is powerful. It is consistent. It makes us stronger, better on all levels. Trusting our inner voice allows us to approach our decisions mindfully and with greater confidence.

Motivated to Live Well – Being Proactive

I want to live a good, productive and positive life. To do that, I have to feel at my best. To do that, I have to eat foods that serve me well – physically, mentally and emotionally. I have to wear clothes that make me feel attractive and energized. I have to spend money wisely. I have to get enough sleep. I have to have fun in ways that I define as fun. I have to interact with others mindfully and positively. Most importantly, I have to spend my time in ways that make me feel balanced in all roles – as wife, mother, daughter, sister, teacher, friend ...

At the end of the day, I don't want to feel that I was led by anyone other than the best version of myself. I don't want to feel that any aspect of my day spun out of control. That's not to say I am under the delusion that I am in control of everything. It is just a mindset. I want to feel proactive, not reactive.

Being proactive means I have a chance to consider, assess and choose based on my values and priorities. Being reactive means I am being pulled, stressed and pressured. Reacting is not good for me or those around me. When I'm reactive, the backlash is ugly – I'm pissed off and totally unpleasant to live with. Thankfully, it doesn't happen often, but when it does, it is highly memorable and we, in the family, are highly motivated to avoid it!

Taking Advantage of the Predictable

Much in life seems predictable. We all have to eat, sleep, work, etc. I don't want to fly by the seat of my pants. I don't feed off that kind of adrenaline. It upsets me to live that way. So, I watch for patterns, both positive and negative. I develop routines, plans of action that set me (and the family) up for success and minimize the potential for the negative, i.e., stress.

The strategies and time management tips are simple: keep an ongoing grocery list, discuss the upcoming week's schedule as a family, have a predictable routine for chores, errands, meal preparation, exercise and rest. The key to keeping stress manageable is doing all those things consistently – even when we don't feel like doing them.

You determine the approach, the path, that helps you feel less stressed. Whatever you choose, consistency is the hardest aspect of maintaining any positive routine. Planning ahead, thinking things through and communicating greatly reduce potential stress – at least most of the time!

Super Woman – Hear Me Roar! (Respectfully)

For the most part, I feel strong, powerful and confident. I feel in charge of most aspects of my life and for the rest of it, I converse with God, ask for support, cry and cope.

Life is life – with all its beauty and tragedy, blessings and challenges. Life is about striving for balance and managing what comes our way in the best ways we can, based on our priorities and life experience up to that moment.

We are all dealing with different strengths and challenges. We are all coming from different places and motivations. Motivations shift, ebb and flow with life. We cannot judge our choices based on anyone else's path. What's good and works for one person may be a total soul sucker for someone else! So what? It is what it is. **No judgment!**

I hate to cook. I love to teach. I taught both kids how to read before they entered kindergarten. I exposed them to the wonders of our city and nature and puppet shows and story times. I read for hours and hours. I learned nursery rhymes and fairy tales. Whatever subject they showed an interest in, we explored. We learned together.

Teaching is my strength and that is where I focused. I did my due diligence to stop judging myself for refusing to make gourmet, organic baby food! The kids never went hungry. I provided healthy'ish options and as soon as they were able, I turned my fabulous teaching skills toward sandwich preparation, the microwave and finally the stove!!

We need to focus awareness, attention and energy on our strengths. We need more compassion, more patience for ourselves and others. We need to feel that we are in charge of our own life. We need to feel **empowered** by our choices – and live accordingly.

One day at a time … one moment at a time …
one breath at a time …

KENDRIA ELLIOTT

46 years old

Single, 3 children

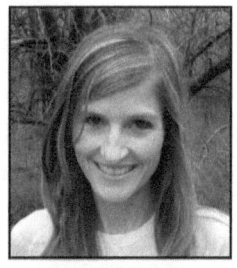

When you look at Kendi Elliott, you see a beautiful, slim woman who, not surprisingly, was a cheerleader in high school and the homecoming queen. What you don't see are the scars from the multiple surgeries she's undergone since being diagnosed with ulcerative colitis in February 2008. What you don't see is the ileostomy bag she has to wear for her small intestine to drain when her internal J-pouch fails. The original J-pouch was formed in 2008; Kendi recently underwent a second seven-hour surgery to construct a new pouch after the initial one failed. Listening to Kendi's story, her rare combination of strength and humility are obvious, along with her unwavering religious faith and a dedication to the yoga and circuit training that not only keep her fit, but thriving.

There are blessings that come out of suffering

I had been taking yoga with Shanna for about five years when all this happened. I lost 35 pounds between February and July 2008. I couldn't even walk up and down stairs by myself. Getting out of the shower, I'd see someone else's body in the mirror. I was taking steroids so my face was all puffy, but my body was skin and bones.

During that same time, I had 12 blood transfusions, and struggled with my hemoglobin counts. I still do. My darkest day was when I went for a transfusion on Friday, had labs on Monday, and the numbers were down – I needed another transfusion. My husband drove me to the hospital and pulled up at the door. I didn't have enough strength to step up the curb.

They did an internal J-pouch construction, but I was too sick to hook it up. I had an ileostomy and external bag for two years; I couldn't drive during that time. I went to see a J-pouch specialist and in March 2010 I had surgery to try and hook it up. That led to an infection, and in May they went back in to fix the damage caused from the infection.

In October 2010 they were finally able to hook up the J-pouch. The next month, in November, I became aware that my husband of 20 years was moving out. He said he didn't want to be married to me anymore and had a new girlfriend. In January 2011, we told the kids and he moved out.

I couldn't drive and was in bed most of the time between 2008 and 2010. When I was finally to the point that I could drive, I would be so nervous and stricken with anxiety – even going to the grocery store. I thought everyone would know I hadn't been to a grocery store in years. Just chit chatting was difficult.

Getting out of bed to go to one of Shanna's classes became one of my biggest accomplishments.

When I started back to yoga, I had to be in child's pose almost all the time. I sobbed the whole time – I couldn't believe what my body had been through. I could do so much before that I couldn't do now. I felt so much younger before. I mourned my old self. I released all that in yoga – I didn't really grieve my own self until I got to yoga.

Shanna would just walk around, put her hand on my back and assure me it was OK. She told me later that it was normal – that yoga clears your mind so emotions can come up.

I did pretty well for almost two years and then got sick again at the end of July 2012. The J-pouch started deteriorating. There was a hole that started leaking stool into my abdomen, and a large abscess. The infection landed me in a wheelchair right before the kids went to school.

This time, I had no husband, my dad had died and my mom doesn't travel much. A girlfriend went to the out-of-town clinic and stayed with me. They unhooked the J-pouch to let it rest and I have an external pouch again now. It's humbling to live with it and go to yoga. It makes noises – it gurgles, air comes out. I think people around me must hear it.

I'm also constantly dealing with inflammation and many times in yoga I can't lay on my stomach. Shanna always has options. She doesn't single me out or make a big deal about it – but she always has an alternative pose. And when she talks about aligning your mind, body and spirit – you can do that even when the body can't do everything you'd want.

I have a very strong faith – I'm a Christian – and my three children and I have a really strong support network. Shanna as a friend is always there. Even if I can't make class, she is always supportive and always encouraging.

Every time I have a surgery, and go back to yoga and circuit classes, I get teary. I feel like I'm back to square one, using three-pound weights. But I need to get stronger and I need to move my joints. I have inflammatory arthritis – it goes with the bowel disease; they're both autoimmune diseases.

I'll always have some kind of joint inflammation but it's so much better to move when you have joint issues. That's the kind of thing

I think about – not a certain aesthetic. I could care less what I look like. I care about how I feel and what I can do to be stronger so if I have another surgery I can sustain life.

Yoga definitely helps. I need to balance life, stress, sleep, diet and medication. It's just like yoga – everything has to be in alignment for you to feel your best. It's tricky. If one thing is off, it's all off.

I've also found that as you transform your body, you transform your mind. And that you don't know just by looking what someone else is going through. They might have struggles with their marriage, their health, finances, aging parents, self-image, children – everyone has something they deal with.

Yet, there are blessings that come out of suffering. I wouldn't change my life. It made me who I am and brought me here. Yoga is the constant – I know it's good for my mind, body and spirit. I couldn't live without yoga.

It's funny. Back in high school, I was best friends with a boy who was homecoming king when I was homecoming queen. He got in touch with me in December of 2012 – he had no idea I'd been sick, divorced and that my dad had died. We began a relationship that month. He knows everything and he's great with it.

Guess what? He does yoga. That's wild.

V. WHAT'S YOUR CURRENCY? COMPASSIONATELY SEEKING *YOUR* MOTIVATION & DRIVE

My motivation is not inspired by "shoulds" or guilt – my first response to that tone is, "Nope, not gonna do it." In fact, I might just do the exact opposite! My approach to teaching is rooted in the idea that most people are not motivated to make positive changes in their life based on guilt or shoulds.

As long as we are alive, we get to practice. We get to explore. We get to decide that this works and this doesn't. We *should* be able to do so without judgment or feeling that we are failures or quitters.

Everyone has different motivating factors. What motivates me certainly doesn't inspire everyone else around me. I have enough evidence in my immediate family to know that I'm quite weird in what spurs my eating choices! Did Drs. Oz or Weil say this food/vitamin is healthy? It smells and looks kind of odd but if they say it's beneficial, then I think I'll try it. It will give me more energy and it is not known to be toxic? Cool! It is high in protein and fiber, low in sugar and contains no dairy (due to a dairy intolerance)? Wow, it sounds perfect!

I currently drink grape chia kombucha tea and have chia, hemp, flax seeds and coconut water as some of the ingredients in my smoothie. Do I imagine I could or should convince anyone else to make those exact same choices? Um, no. Hardly.

I view my health as an experiment. Can my lifestyle outsmart my genes? Can I have a high quality of life into my 80s and beyond? Can I age well? Can I be a healthy example for my children and break the cycle of my grandparents and father?

I don't know. I really don't know. But I am highly motivated to try. I've seen the alternative and it does not appeal to me.

But, Why to Such a Degree?

I think there are some who look at my food and exercise choices as extreme. Truly, they don't feel extreme … they feel enthusiastic!

Firstly, I find everyday life far more pleasant by eating healthy and exercising. Secondly, and this seems like such a strange connection, but my food choices are highly influenced by being the granddaughter of immigrants. I have so many memories wrapped up around their relationship with food and watching them with a foreigner's eyes (my own).

I listened to their stories. I saw how their past affected their present. They struggled and lost so much. For significant times in their lives, they had absolutely nothing. They were hated and abandoned by their neighbors, simply for being themselves – for being Jewish. Everything was taken from them, everything – unimaginable kinds of everything.

In spite of so much going against them, they survived. They started over and led productive lives. They created families filled with love. And, like the rest of us, their past influenced the choices they made.

Being focused on eating healthy and exercising were a totally foreign concept – my eating choices were on the edge of bizarre – and insulting to their experiences. How could I deprive myself in such ways? How could I explain that I didn't at all feel deprived?

They wanted to celebrate and revel in the foods that were readily available and affordable! The rest of the consequences be damned. Sickness impacted their lives but not in a way that demonstrated any awareness of the connection between their choices and their ailments. What I saw as suffering, they saw as normal aging and expected.

My Baba would have a stomachache and request to be driven to the grocery store to purchase chicken livers. I have story upon story like that. Much of the time, my thoughts were, "Say what??!!" How are chicken livers, pastrami, or herring a cure for a stomachache or a cold? Baba would say to me, "You don't know everything, Shanna! Don't judge me!"

I didn't understand. I didn't get it. But, today I do. Now, I can see. None of those things were meant to be a cure, they were meant to be a comfort. She was right in telling me to just shut the hell up! I was being disrespectful. I was judging. I did not understand the connection or the intention.

I was born into privilege. I was born in a comparatively safe country. I have always been surrounded by love and support. I have never gone hungry or truly without. Compared to all that they lived through and witnessed, I am rich beyond measure.

I am not driven by fear for survival – I take that for granted. Up to this moment, I have had my health, my safety – mostly a peaceful mind! I don't need to celebrate at every meal in order to manage the unimaginable memories of the past or to make up for them.

I am aware of my family history, the legacy I was born into and I feel responsible to it. I feel responsible to take my advantages and live certain aspects of my life differently than they did ... because I can. Those values drive and positively motivate my choices every single day.

Now, all that being said, are my mother, sister, children driven by these same things? No. Does that mean they have any less love or appreciation for their past? Absolutely not! It just isn't a part of their psyche in the same way. Even if it were, chances are it wouldn't be motivating. It would just be guilt-inducing or some other negative quality. Who needs that?!

My values are driven by how I interpret the world. I saw a connection between all sorts of things and I don't love food enough to enjoy the benefits. I am grateful and appreciative for food. I am grateful and appreciative for the conveniences of quickly prepared meals. My personal choices are no hardship or deprivation ... and in their own way – my choices are a celebration.

Respect Your Motivations

We are all varied and what motivates us is equally varied. A primary incentive for your food choices might be taste, comfort or familiarity. Those are perfectly valid and should be respected.

Everyone defines happiness and life satisfaction differently. My father might have lived longer with different food and lifestyle choices but he also would have been miserable along the way (and a total bear to live with). His currency, what motivated him, was completely different than mine.

Once we were eating in a buffet restaurant together and he looked at my mostly empty plate, became irritated and said we were not restaurant compatible. He was right. What and where he loved to eat, I did not enjoy.

Once Dad tried going to the gym with me, but then announced in the middle of the weights area that he had absolutely no interest in getting bulky. I just silently giggled because the man was so visibly strong and bulky. I never knew he was self-conscious about it. So, we found ways to spend time together that were mutually agreeable and avoided irritants.

"Shoulds" Won't Stick for Long

Knowing what motivates us is part of the journey of self-discovery and absolutely vital to success in all areas of our life. Most of us cannot endlessly do something out of obligation without it eating away at our insides – regardless if it is a job, a diet or anything else. "Shoulds" can start us on a path but they won't provide long-term motivation.

When I was experimenting with different professions on my path of career discovery, occupations just wouldn't stick. I bounced from job to job and business idea. My father started to wonder if I was a quitter – which was especially difficult to discuss. I knew it wasn't true and he didn't really believe that I was a quitter. But, we were both perplexed. What the hell was my problem?

I learned – just because you can do something well does not mean it is what you are supposed to be doing … long-term. It just demonstrates that you have discipline and a work ethic – admirable but no guarantee of happiness or true success.

I've been teaching yoga and fitness to adults since 2005 and I am more motivated and inspired by my career today than at the beginning. Each year is as though I am just now coming into my groove. Each year I fall in love with it all over again. Teaching has stuck and elevates my soul. I get paid to share my passion.

I knew I wasn't a quitter. I just had to have faith and not quit on myself. I had to be okay with others judging me (especially my dad). I couldn't give up on myself or what I discovered was one of my highest values: I craved living a positive and purposeful life that made me feel passionate and excited.

Start, Stop, Reassess

Until going through the process of starting, stopping and reassessing, I had no idea what I really valued. Initially, I thought earning money was most important or doing something with my B.A. in Psychology. Figuring out what mattered most to me **required** the process of exploration and elimination.

It wasn't money or status. Along the way, I figured out I was driven by feeling helpful, passionate and appreciated. Students showing up for my classes, expressing enthusiasm, inspires and motivates me to keep learning and doing my best. I equate this personal experience to others' self-discovery about eating and exercise.

Just because someone has tried a thousand different diets and started/stopped an exercise routine a gazillion times does NOT mean they are quitters or failures

They just haven't found the right method that speaks to them; they haven't figured out their personal currency – their specific motivation that will drive them long-term. With each experience, they know a little bit more about themselves and what motivates or drains them. They are that much closer to figuring out what fits and matters most. There is probably an exercise out there that suits but is impacted by cost, convenience, intensity, environment, or community of people who show up.

Don't give up on yourself. If you have struggled and are yearning for a healthier lifestyle, then keep searching. Your right exercise, class, teacher is out there ... and is waiting for you.

Potential Motivator: Discovering YOUR Right Community

I know that feeling connected to fellow classmates is a big factor for many of my students. Most of my classes are held in a community center. Oftentimes, there are kids running down the halls or parents talking right outside the door. Room temperature might be too cold or too hot – and we work on finding a temperature that most can agree on! But the place fits the bill because none of those qualities are anyone's highest currency.

Most students enter my classes with the knowledge that there are people who look forward to and expect to see them. In turn, they look forward to visiting with their: yoga peeps, Pilates peeps, and/or circuit peeps. Strangers become friends, tuned in to one another's lives. That connection to community keeps them motivated to attend regularly. That connection to community transforms class time to something far greater and significant than a fitness goal alone. Community becomes integral to the process of living healthy. (More on Community in Ch. IX. Learning & Gripping)

Potential Motivator: Discovering YOUR Right Teacher

As a teacher, I am thrilled and honored to be a motivator and a supporter. I'm happy to do everything I can to assist on their journey. Part of that process is assisting students in discovering their currency. I am not everyone's right teacher. If someone is looking for a high intensity, intricate yoga "workout" that requires sweat, I will never see them again.

People pre-enroll for my classes. I have the opportunity to speak with many before they ever try a class. I introduce myself and talk about my style (intentional, methodical, step-by-step approach). I ask about what inspired them to sign up. What are they hoping to get out of the class?

In this process, I am finding out about their expectations and simultaneously giving them an idea of what to expect from me. I get to encourage them to be patient and compliment them for choosing to try the class. I assure them that if it turns out not to be the right fit, no worries, I will not be offended. They don't have to worry about bumping into me outside of class. Fear and self-doubt are minimized. They can walk into class with more confidence and ease. It is a wonderful advantage that many teachers don't have.

Potential Motivator: Giving Yourself Some Credit!

For someone to continue showing up for my classes inspires me. No matter how dedicated, each student is overcoming an obstacle or a set of obstacles to be present. It is my job to show up. I am getting paid. I don't have to justify my reason to anyone. I am doing what I love.

The students have to justify their energy, mood, time, cost, traffic and any other tasks demanding their attention. They have to justify all this to themselves as well as to their loved ones. They have to stop whatever it is they are currently doing to go exercise. For many people, this is no casual decision.

Most individuals don't give themselves enough credit. Just because exercise and eating healthy are "shoulds" in life does not mean that you haven't earned tremendous kudos by getting yourself to class or making healthful choices. Continuing, staying, on a healthy journey is a constant choice.

If exercise is not something you like to do, you are incredible for choosing it anyway. Doing things you don't want to do, simply because they are good for you, is true discipline and a highly underrated accomplishment.

Potential Motivator: Finding What Makes YOU Feel Successful

Who hasn't struggled? We all struggle. Some people's struggles are simply more apparent and others are more successfully hidden. Losing weight (if that's a goal) and keeping it off are some of the hardest things in life to do. It means changing some of your most personal and frequent habits. The change has to last forever to be lauded "successful." Setbacks are public … totally exposed.

Keeping weight off means overcoming and managing constant temptation at every single meal. It means being vulnerable at every gathering or dining out experience; potentially with family, friends and strangers watching how much you eat and judging your choices. Everyone has their own theories of *appropriate* or *healthy* food portions and body size. Observers judge from that viewpoint.

People judge without putting a microscope to their own, less visible struggles. Do not give that kind of energy space within you. Forbid it from entering your psyche. Put up a stop sign. Put up a hand and say, "You are not welcome here!"

Surround yourself with supportive peers, supportive thoughts. Let's put it this way: does the alternate strategy feel successful? Would it really hurt to be nicer to yourself – with your thoughts, words and deeds?

The journey is hard enough without additional pressure. Give yourself credit for all the choices that make you feel good, strong and capable. Give yourself a break from the rest. Self-punishment on top of struggle is counterproductive.

Focus on your successes! I assure you, there are many. Make a mental or written list of all your wins at the end of each day. Read it – as many times as it takes for you to go to sleep feeling more positive than negative about your day. No one else has to define them as wins – you are the one making the list! You know what you overcame and food is not exclusive to this list. Did you almost yell at someone for making an incompetent choice and then choose to respond respectfully? Win! Score!

One of my kids (and I won't say who) used to be quite the tattler. So that said person would not become friendless at the age of six, I suggested recording a tally in a small notebook for every time tattling was a temptation. At the end of the day, we went over the tallies and discussed all the specific situations. Every tally was a WIN! We celebrated.

Keep a tally of your wins. Honor your successes. Share them or not. What can it possibly hurt?

You are a Practicer & You are Allowed to Evolve

It is hard to keep self-doubt at bay. We all have strengths that boost our confidence and situations that bring our fears and anxiety to the forefront. Do not be led by fear and do not give up on yourself. You are not a quitter nor a failure. You are a **practicer**. You are giving things a go and seeing if they stick.

Changing your mind about what suits does not define you as wishy-washy or flaky. We learn as much about ourselves by discovering things we don't like as those we do. As difficult as it was in the moment, I am grateful for all the jobs I discovered that don't fit me. I have experiences to speak from and absolute gratitude for individuals who make a living doing jobs I can't abide.

Thank you to teachers of children. Thank you, God, for all teachers of children! Thank you to sales people, social workers and therapists. Thank you to professional organizers. Thank you to creative people everywhere. Thank you to people who like to cook. Thank **YOU** for whatever it is you are doing that is most likely under-appreciated.

Be kind to yourself and your efforts. Showing up with a willing spirit to give a healthier lifestyle a try (even or especially if it is the gazillionth time) is an accomplishment unto itself. Holla Holla!!

Consciously Ask: What Matters Most to YOU … Right Now?

Finding the motivation and drive to make positive, **sustainable** health changes has to be congruent with your values. It means consciously asking what matters most to YOU – right now? What is your currency? It doesn't have to fit anyone else's definition.

Are you looking to increase energy, decrease stress, lose weight or something else entirely?

If no physical activity is all that pleasurable, are there any that are palatable? Would you be interested in trying to do one of them for five minutes daily? Can you identify one food you eat habitually that holds no emotional attachment? Can you replace it with one healthier alternative? Do you notice if any of these choices make a positive, worthwhile difference to your energy – or have a positive impact on your goal?

There is no judgment; it is all an exploration and experiment. Start something again or something new with the attitude that it is just a test-drive. If you are sharing this news with others – then say it as such. You are making no promises or absolute resolutions. You have every right to just try … and see.

As you find strategies that work for you, internal motivation grows. Temptation ebbs and flows. As you accumulate more positive evidence, choosing better gets easier. Not easy, just easier. Choices are made with greater awareness. A growing cycle of, "When I chose this healthier option, the positive result was this and the positive result was worth the choice."

There is no dissatisfaction or deprivation. Over time and with practice, making decisions you define as "good" becomes part of your overall routine. Understanding your personal motivations leads you to feeling more empowered on all levels – physically, mentally and emotionally. Feeling empowered by your choices leads to increased drive to continue living life with greater awareness.

It is all a process. It is all a practice. Becoming the best version of you is a constant exploration, a journey. It might as well be as enjoyable as possible!

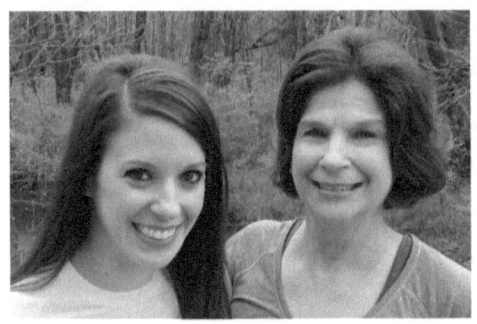

LAUREN CASON
30 years old
Married, no children

BARBARA CASON
60 years old
Married, four children

One look at Lauren Cason and you might think she'd fit in at any gym in the country. Look again. Lauren doesn't like gyms. However, this former dancer does like exercising, and she's found a place where she feels right at home – Shanna's circuit training, Pilates and yoga classes. Speaking of home, the woman right next to Lauren during class is her mother. Barbara Cason is an amazing role model for her four daughters and everyone around her. A master gardener, Barbara radiates energy. A conversation with this enthusiastic duo is its own kind of exercise – imagine a Ping-Pong game and keep your eye on the ball!

Keep going! Keep trying! Try something new. Just keep going.

Lauren: I danced in high school and was in my best shape then. But in college I didn't do anything. I moved home, and saw they were going to have a yoga class at the rec center.

Barbara: Has it already been seven years?

L: We didn't know anything about Shanna until after we had enrolled – we took both the hatha and power yoga classes.

B: I hadn't done any organized exercise until then. Now, I go to yoga to relax. Mentally and physically, it's wonderful for de-stressing and I think that's important. You can really leave the world behind, and that helps a lot.

L: I have never been a fitness buff or a gym person, but from the very beginning I liked yoga. You use your own body to help you get in shape. I really like that it involves flexibility and strength since I danced for so many years.

B: And, in your 60s and beyond, there's an increase in falls – and falls can really take people down. Every time you fall, there's a risk you'll break something. Yoga is a gentle way to keep going. There are times when I feel tired and don't want to go to class, but I do feel so much better afterwards. At my age, I'm trying not to lose flexibility. If I miss a couple of sessions, I really notice – the yoga helps me keep arthritis at bay. I need to keep these old joints moving!

L: We both just feel better when we do something. The first time I did Crow pose, I was like, *Whoa!* I had no idea that I was able to do something that you usually see in magazines. And Shanna always mixes things up – she knows how to work a different muscle group each time. I also like the discipline of having the classes pre-scheduled since I'm not one to work out on my own. I enjoy the variety that Shanna's classes offer.

B: And we know to never really assume what someone in class is able to do.

L: That's right! I don't like running – my body hurts afterwards. And I think gyms are kind of intimidating. I've never known how to use the equipment properly.

B: The gym is full of torture devices without someone to show you how to use them properly. The treadmill feels like a hamster wheel!

L: If you're not attentive, you can do it wrong, you lose the form and you can hurt yourself. So many people don't know what proper form is.

B: With Shanna, even though it's a group, she makes it feel one on one, making modifications if you have issues.

L: Like my hips and quads are really flexible and Shanna is always trying to get me to work them, in the right form!

B: I work with a bunch of master gardeners – some people 20 years older than I am are in better shape! They're out there, digging the dirt, moving it. A lot of them are older but they're in really good shape and they're all active. They don't say, "I hurt. I'm gonna quit." They're part of the Greatest Generation. They get up and fight again.

L: My mom is definitely a role model for us – except when we were kids she would say, "No dessert for breakfast!" and then she would eat it! But when it comes to food, I think it's about balance. I'm kind of a foodie. I love to cook and try new recipes and go out and try new restaurants.

B: If you cut out everything until life isn't fun anymore, what's the point?

L: But I don't eat like that every day! For the most part, I try to eat relatively heathfully. On a daily basis, you do what you're supposed to do. I indulge more on weekends than during the week, but it's all about balance.

B: We don't know what tomorrow holds, so as long as we're here, we might as well be in as good a shape as possible. Keep going! Keep trying! Try something new. Get in good shape now – exercise can only be good for your aging and balance. I want to be like my 104-year-old aunt. You know what she says? "If I fall down, I get back up." I want to be like that.

VI. TWEAKING & TREATING

I am in charge of our finances; my husband is allowed to see whatever he wants but he is not allowed to pay the bills nor enter anything into Quicken®. Money is MY domain. It keeps me in check. Sitting down every day to monitor our accounts prevents me from overspending and gives me assurance that our goals are still attainable. I find managing our finances comforting. It gives me a sense of security in this unpredictable world.

I've created a "financial map." It is organized by year with all our ages and kids' school grade levels. Below each year are bullets of major events. This way I can see that my daughter will be graduating high school during the same year that my son will be having his bar mitzvah during the same year that the house may need painting. The financial map has been a very helpful tool, minimizing being caught off guard by things we know are coming but still have a tendency to creep up.

I review this map regularly. Some might call it a budget but my bossy side would reply, "I don't create budgets." I look at our current life patterns, assess our goals and create a map that sets us up for success. We discuss the map as a family so we are all on the same page – on a joint mission.

I don't place expectations or obligations on us that we have never previously accomplished or only accomplished "BK" – before kids. Having a financial map helps us figure out what matters most to us right now and for the years to come.

Where would we like to see ourselves in the years ahead? What big home maintenance projects will be needed and when? How can we prepare? What choices do we need to make today to help the kids pursue their dreams?

What are the predictable life expenses that we should be aware of such as braces, wisdom teeth and bar/bat mitzvahs? Can we plan as much as possible for the years to come and then surrender to faith that we will figure out how to handle and afford those events we can't predict?

Values shift with time and age. So, we reassess. Knowing what we value, having a fair idea of what's coming, assists and motivates us in making mindful choices today. It also gives us ideas of how and when to splurge. Splurging, treating oneself, is absolutely essential for the sweetness of life. We have been given this gift called life; it is our responsibility, privilege and blessing to live fully.

We need to treat ourselves and be aware of the gifts of being alive. We need to restore, replenish, renew – whatever word speaks to you. We need to make deposits into our internal bank account so that we are fueled for the demands of day-to-day life.

We cannot make constant demands on our self-discipline, receive no reward and expect to stay on plan. We also cannot purchase everything to our heart's desire and expect to have money left for the mortgage. The key, as always, is balance.

A Health Map

The same rules or techniques apply to living a healthier lifestyle. To begin a "Health Map," one of the first questions I ask any new client is, "Tell me about your typical day." If they don't have a typical day in regards to food and activity level, then I ask about the factors that seem to prevent it. Is it a lack of interest or appeal? Is it not having any idea of where to start? How would they most like my help?

Then we discuss the foods that they love. I assure them that this is a "no judgment zone." I want to know things as they are right now. I want to know the foods they most value so we can keep them in the map. I call this gorge protection, also known as overspending protection, also known as preventing overdoing in any capacity.

What foods are they highly attached to? What would make them sad or resentful to never or rarely eat again? And, what foods are they merely eating out of convenience?

Just as proximity is a huge factor in finding the right exercise venue, so is convenience when it comes to eating healthy. If healthy versus non-healthy options are equally convenient, then chances are we will choose better on a regular basis. If they are equally appealing … all the better.

Another early question is in regards to energy level. Do they feel like they have enough energy to accomplish their daily tasks/goals? Or, do they run short of energy frequently? If they feel low on energy, is it at a predictable time of day? What tends to precipitate the dip? What do they do about it? What is the quality of their sleep? Do they have a regular sleep schedule?

Feeling that we have enough energy to accomplish what matters most to us (on a regular basis) has a direct impact on our sense of accomplishment and self-confidence. It is key to feeling successful in all aspects of our life.

If weight loss is a goal, is there an ideal size/weight? When was the last time in their life that they **lived at** (not reached) that size/weight? How is their life different today? How would the quality of their life improve by making all the necessary changes to sustain that weight/size?

No Big Overhaul Allowed

The initial interview process is fascinating. People typically come in tense with a vibe that says, "Here we go again, I totally suck at this." Then, we start discussing what truly motivates them. We move through the questions and their attitude shifts. I ask, "What do you think about tweaking this one meal in this small way?" They invariably tell me, "Oh, I can totally do that!"

I would never suggest nor recommend a complete overhaul of someone's life. For most people, dramatic change is not sustainable – not with money, time management, food or anything else. We are creatures of habit. Those habits are sources of familiarity and comfort. For most of us, big change is scary, stressful, unnecessary and most often unsuccessful.

Living and maintaining a presumed ideal weight that clients initially say they want would not guarantee a happy or balanced life. If clients are really determined to have a goal weight then I almost always shoot out an alternate number and include a range of several pounds. I ask if they ever sustained that range for any length of time and how was their life in that time. The number might not be what they expected but the typical response is positive. Then, I explain my strategy of tweaking.

Tweaking is painless. Tweaking is small adjustments, almost unnoticeable, that over time result in huge changes and are far less shocking and stressful. Tweaking prevents gorging and allows for treats.

Tweaking is a positive, empowered way to decrease spending and save money, lose pounds, have more energy or affect any other currency. Tweaking means less significant setbacks. An attitude of tweaking allows for forgiveness and positive self-talk.

We want to be the best version of ourselves – not the version someone else defines. Maintenance is work but it shouldn't be an enormous struggle. We can't white knuckle our way through life. If nothing else, we would be miserable company.

We are not trying to get through any one meal or event. It is meal after meal, event after event, until we die. It is the human version of forever. We can choose to feel agonized by the process. However, I think **agony is our inner language, our inner voice begging for our life to be different**. We can choose to be militant about our choices but that seems severe and unnecessary. Tweaking mitigates the lure of extremes. As we witness the positive impact of tweaking, we can acknowledge that improvements are occurring – possibly slowly and steadily but happening, nonetheless. Tweaking becomes a part of our **lifestyle**.

Balance is Not a Fixed State

My goal is to strive for balance in all things. Balance is not a fixed state of being. We are not perfectly even. We are not physically symmetrical. We are NOT robots – all the more so when in movement. Our body responds and adapts to keeping us upright as much as possible. Wobbling is a necessary ability and response. I repeat: wobbling, making micro-adjustments, is a necessary ability and applies to **EVERYTHING**.

Staying balanced in a yoga pose **requires** micro movements, tweaking and constant adjustments – from the soles of our feet all the way up the body. We balance in stillness for a moment and then subtle movements occur in the foot, knee or itchy nose! Sometimes we have to put a foot down or exit the pose. Given the chance to reset, we typically return to a stronger and steadier stance.

Every new student (and even some not so new) says, "My balance is terrible." "I suck at balance." All I think is, how are you measuring? What are your criteria? Are you supposed to hold a pose indefinitely, never needing a break, never having to MOVE?? Is this expectation realistic or fair? Is there any successful part of your life where the same would hold true? **Are we absolutely PERFECT at anything?**

What makes someone "good" at balance anyway? Do students think I am good at balance? Are they watching me? Because I tweak and reset a lot. Every day is different. Sometimes, I am a little steadier. Other days, I am wobbling like crazy, laughing, and letting everyone know not to make me their focal point. No one pose on any particular day defines my ability to balance or practice yoga.

I enjoy the challenge of practicing balance poses. "Practicing" being the optimal word. Sometimes – for some moments – I can control the micro movements; I tap into sensations of strength, precision ... absolute awareness. It feels beautiful and empowering. Other times, I can barely get my butt up, forget to breathe and crack up as I fall out.

Ultimately, I expect to come out of a pose. Sometimes, it is a graceful exit and other times ... it is ... indescribable!

Perfection is NOT the Goal

Yoga/exercise is the only area of my life that I can easily enter with the attitude of humor and forgiveness. All is okay. All is well. Perfection is not the goal. No matter what, I always feel better post practice.

Part of my learning and life practice is to take that attitude with me to other endeavors "off the yoga mat." I am working on it. I am working on it. And life has a way of providing plenty of opportunities to practice!

If we all allow ourselves permission to put the darn foot down; however ungracefully ... smile, give ourselves a moment of awareness to reset, the return ascent is pretty painless.

Living at a healthy weight and size is a constant process, a constant striving for balance, requiring daily decisions within the minutia of life. We are never done. There is no "cure" or "perfect." Our needs, interests and values change as our life changes. It is *NECESSARY* to wobble, tweak and reset.

Each day provides opportunity to begin anew, with the life experience accumulated thus far. Each day we are a little bit further into this experiment named our life and we know a little bit more about ourselves.

It is also yet another day to be faced with many of the same decisions and temptations **over and over again**. As Dr. Phil would say, "How's it workin' for ya?" Is your current strategy creating a successful feeling in your life? Are you requiring perfection as your definition of healthy so therefore why bother, or are you allowing yourself room to wobble, to tweak and to treat?

Treats!

Are you providing yourself opportunities to restore, replenish and renew – sans guilt? I eat a small dessert two to three times daily. I love dessert, look forward to it and feel only pure pleasure eating it! I relax every evening with my favorite television shows – rarely highbrow! I take a 15-30 minute nap almost daily between teaching classes and prior to picking up the kids from school. I sleep in at least one day on the weekend. I take fitness/yoga classes up to six times weekly – a total mind/body restorer. In the last couple of years, we've been able to afford twice a month house cleaning – and that is a HUGE treat for the entire family! Since my feet are seen and stared at daily, I feel totally justified in getting a monthly pedicure. Even though I love my job, I have learned over the years that vacations are necessary! So, I schedule time off around the kids' school breaks.

In what ways are you treating yourself … daily, weekly, monthly, annually? Do you recognize how critical those treats are to living a balanced life … to feeling at your best and **giving** your best to all those around you? We can't life a positive, productive life without treats. Just like everything else, we get to create our own definition of what that entails.

Life is not about striving for perfection or *skinny*. It's about living the best possible life each and every day. It's about striving to improve and learn more along the way.

Attaining *skinny* has no real fulfillment unless it is partnered with overall life satisfaction. Skinny does not necessarily mean healthy. Skinny does not mean you have perfect balance. Skinny does not guarantee that you have the energy to do, accomplish or strive toward your dreams. Skinny does not mean you have a superb attitude or beautiful self-talk. Skinny does not mean that you are flexible or strong. Skinny does not mean you have all of your shit together or think you are perfect. *Skinny is just a SIZE. Skinny is just a NUMBER.*

Go for TWEAKS, allow for TREATS!

JULIE CHESIS
49 years old
Married, two daughters, two sons

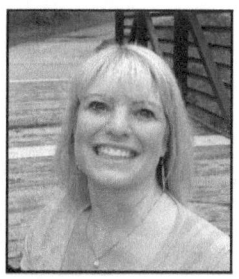

Ask five people to describe Julie Chesis and they'll tell you she's fun. Vivacious. The life of the party. Cheerful, friendly, outgoing, warm, lovely, kind and loving. The word "shy" will not come up. "Reserved" will not be mentioned. And "terrified" certainly won't be on the list. Yet, despite her genuine, enthusiastic, hostess-with-the-mostest personality, Julie pulls back in one area. She is scared to talk about her weight loss and years of steadfast workouts with Shanna. Why? She's not sure. Maybe it's a fear of failure. Maybe it just feels too personal.

This time, I did something I'd never done before

I don't feel private and scary about anything else – ask me about my sex life, my kiddos, anything. I'll tell you more than you want to know. But this is really personal and it freaks me out. It's a little mind blowing. My friends know I've lost weight but I haven't told them the specifics. Maybe it's fear of failure? I don't know. So, to be sharing all this seems kind of weird, but here goes.

I first started doing this April 12, 2011. I started because it was 2½ years before I'd turn 50 and I wanted to see where I could be health-wise, weight-wise, and strength-wise before I reached 50. I had heard Shanna used to be a personal trainer, and I thought, here's a lovely, compassionate woman. I'll ask her.

Unbeknownst to me, she wasn't doing private personal training. But she did it with me and it worked. I knew nothing about the correct way to do things – I was not in good shape and I would not have had the stamina or accountability to do it on my own.

But, when we started, there was nothing hardcore. There was no yelling at me. It wasn't easy but it was doable. "Can you do one more rep?" Sure, I can do one more. Then she saw what I could do, and she'd have me do something else … she always made me feel like I made progress.

We'd talk afterwards and she'd give me tips. But she didn't tell me what to eat and what not to eat – what I must do. She just gave me little hints, advice, tips on what to do. Shanna didn't break out a measuring tape and measure my thighs. But my thighs felt better in my jeans.

It took a while and the weight came off slowly, but I lost two dress sizes by October.

Now, I'm clearly more mindful about my eating, but I won't say I don't eat fattening things. I'm more mindful, but I don't deny myself. If I want a bowl of ice cream, because that's my favorite thing in the world, I eat a bowl of ice cream. The thing is, now I'm burning calories. I also eat what I want in smaller portions – smaller goodies and expending calories, that's how I keep it off. The key part is I continue to move and hopefully always will.

I couldn't work out with others when I started. It gave me courage to have Shanna help me privately at first. Now I can't even imagine doing it without the other ladies.

The big thing for me is accountability – I'm accountable to Shanna and the others in the class, sure, but it's more important to be personally accountable. I put the classes on my calendar and I'm accountable to show up.

After I lost the weight, most of the things in my closet didn't fit and I had to totally shop. That was one of the hardest things for me. I'd lost weight and gained before and had lots of different sizes in my closet. But this time, I did something I'd never done before. I got rid of all my clothes that didn't fit. This was huge for me. I considered storing them – before, I always just left them in my closet. Instead, I totally got rid of them. Totally. Bags and bags of clothes.

I still don't know that I'm confident about that – it was the hardest decision I ever made. But when I started, it felt brave. And then going shopping was unbelievably fun. It was way more exciting than I thought it would be. Shopping had always been a kind of sad, disappointing thing – even though I could always find some cute things. And there are always shoes! But I actually went out and found pants that were cute and jeans that fit! I could tuck in a shirt and it looked cute! That's just off-the-chart mind-boggling.

Packing for my last trip was a blast. Before, it would have been, "Oh, great. I've got to find six outfits." This time, I could stand in my closet knowing everything fit! I like my outfits. I like my clothes. It's an astounding feeling.

Four years ago, we went to Israel as a family. I couldn't walk Masada. This summer, I'm going back and the group leader said, "We walk on average three miles a day," and I said, "That's great!" I'm ready for it.

I'll tell you something. I don't celebrate my birthday. It's an oddity in my personality. I stopped at 30. It's not just not having a party. I don't celebrate at all. But, this year, I might. I'm thinking about having a party. I'm feeling better about it. And that's because of all this. You know how I feel?

Like this is my year. This is my year.

VII. AUTHENTIC MEASURES OF SUCCESS

In our initial assessment, I never take a client's measurements nor do I take photos. I just can't get myself to do it. I don't believe in judging accomplishments or success by any number nor do I want to get hung up on an image. I am not confident that I'll ever be able to remeasure in the exact same spot with any tools easily available, such as a soft measuring tape or a body fat caliper. It is far too easy to be inaccurate, especially when looking for incremental changes. I feel badly if results are disappointing AND the client is left feeling dejected. As far as photos, I don't want to give a client any more reason to feel bad about where they perceive they currently are with so-called "before" images.

In my early years of personal training, I let the client set the intention and goals. I thought it was what I was supposed to do. Unbeknownst to me, I was entering their vicious, well-tested, unsuccessful cycle AND reaffirming their negative self-fulfilling prophecy. Whoa!

Our sessions always started out on a good note. We assessed their goals, took physical measurements, created a plan and met weekly to work out. I suggested they keep a food log. A couple pounds lost, half an inch here or there gone. I felt obligated to ask how their previous week went in regards to food and activity level. I thought I wasn't an authentic trainer unless I also focused on typical, measurable results.

After a short while, numbers would spiral. Measurements were erratic, not moving fast enough or in the wrong direction. I wondered to myself, *what the hell is happening?* The clients' dramatic shifts and disappointments caught me off guard and I felt their angst. But I was only with them for an hour once or twice a week. What were our workouts really supposed to accomplish?

Personal training income was paying for my yoga training. Once I paid off the expense, I left. I felt drained and unhelpful. I was not cut out for the emotional and volatile ride.

Several years later, a wonderful friend, Julie Chesis, asked if I would help her get into shape. Inside, I thought, UGH! I like Julie but what if she ends up feeling disappointed? Our lives are intertwined and she won't want to be around me. So, I said we would talk about it – a wonderfully convenient delay tactic.

I sat at my computer contemplating; this woman is fun and positive – an absolute delight to hang out with. I have the knowledge, ability and time. There has to be a way for this process to feel successful, regardless of any so-called "results." I decided that I would create the intention for our time together. I would dictate how results would be measured. I would do this for her and anyone else who might come my way – and then they did!

Shanna's Rules of Engagement

Rule #1: No measurements, no food logs, no scale ... NADA!

Demanding to know all that data is belittling and shaming. If someone wants to get on a scale, so be it. They want to share a number with me? Completely fine, but I am not intruding. I truly do not care. I don't measure success that way.

Over the years, I've learned that the following types of students gravitate toward me:

a) The total beginner who is intimidated or overwhelmed by the process
b) The tryer who has attempted many times and "failed"
c) The practitioner who appreciates detailed focus on alignment and safety

I don't draw the die-hard workout student. Therefore, my approach should not be as such. Someone asking for my help is probably overcoming a history of self-defeating thoughts and fear. I will not add more pressure to their journey. I want them to feel successful and motivated to continue on a healthier path – for their body, mind and soul.

Rule #2: No dramatic overhaul demanded or encouraged.

Maintaining a consistent workout regimen is a big change for many individuals. Initially, that will be the only goal. Once working out feels natural to their lifestyle, we **can** reassess and add other areas to tweak. Reassessment is at the client's discretion and initiation. Since I don't draw the die-hard student, my focus can be – and is – on providing a physically as well as emotionally safe environment. A student gets an "A" for consistently showing up!

Rule #3 – Clarify the definition of "measurable results" and success.

Success is quickly noticing an increase in energy and overall wellbeing – especially apparent on workout days. After about a month, I expect a demonstrable increase in strength and stamina. I encourage them to lift heavier weights and/or do more repetitions than when we began. I expect them to complain – in a humorous way! I expect them to feel more aware in their body and ask more detailed questions about their physical alignment. Voila! Initially, those are the measurable results that I'm seeking.

In time, clothing might feel a little looser. Pounds and inches may be lost. If that is desired and it occurs then we celebrate! But, it will not be my focus. **When starting to work out, pounds may actually be gained.** Muscle weighs more than fat but clothing could fit the same or looser. Muscle takes up less space!

I consider it quite an accomplishment every time I have to purchase additional sets of heavier weights for my circuit ladies! We celebrate and brag about it frequently!

FIVE ADDITIONAL MEASURES OF SUCCESS

1. Improved Awareness

Once students get over the newness of exercising, my main (and ongoing) goal involves improving their sensory awareness. Students frequently say that they hear my cues in their head as they go about their day. They notice that they stand taller and feel stronger. They feel less fragile and less vulnerable to injury. They maneuver in physical tasks with greater awareness. Overall, they move more mindfully. It is a complete paradigm shift. It is a shift that they did not expect to experience at this age or phase in their life.

They notice the positive impact on so many levels and share their stories. Some measure taller at the doctor, pack heavier bags at the grocery store, find it easier to rake the leaves or shovel snow and on and on. Hearing their observations, witnessing their transformation is incredibly rewarding. It fuels my passion and my mission!

I consider myself in a battle with disconnection. The majority of students come to me with the exact same patterns (no matter their physical shape). They are moderately aware of muscles that are easy to see. Biceps and quadriceps (front thigh muscles) tend to be strong'ish. However, triceps, back muscles, glutes and hamstrings are all weak from underuse or lack of awareness.

Students feel tension around their neck, lower back or both because their body is not being used efficiently. Strength and awareness in their front half is not balanced with their back half. The top half of their body is disassociated from their bottom half. And, they have absolutely no idea what the heck I am talking about!

It all starts out as a foreign language. I ask them to feel sensations that they have never been aware of or given name. I ask them to use their body as a unit, an integrated machine – to feel breath and strength everywhere simultaneously. I explain that every action has an emphasis but no muscle works in isolation. A bicep curl uses the entire body with an emphasis on the bicep. *Why do I have to engage my thighs and butt if I am doing a bicep curl?!!* Because I said so.

Initially, students feel confounded by the process because they can't lift as much weight or do as many reps as they think they *should* be able to do. They also realize that they can't check out – their brains are a required element in the process. Over time, as students tune in to their alignment, regardless of how much weight they are lifting, they feel stronger – **everywhere**. Muscle tone becomes more visible throughout their body.

Their mind and entire body participate in every single movement. As time passes, it is very likely that they **will** lift more weight or do more reps than they ever did previously. But the priority – and what has greater significance – is the internal evidence of improved awareness and sensation. Body within body is connected. Mind and body are connected. Quality over quantity. The rest is just a number and inconsequential in the big scheme of things.

Moving and living with improved awareness is truly life changing. It makes every workout more effective. It makes every movement more successfully accomplished and less likely to cause damage. It means we possess tools to make every decision with greater knowledge. Possessing and refining those tools can impact how and what we eat, how we interact with other human beings, how we spend money and how we use our time and energy. Enhanced awareness can impact EVERYTHING – if we so choose. Inner awareness is our most vital, lifelong teacher. When we cease to live disconnected from our physical selves, we live more connected within. We realize that EVERYTHING in our life, every decision we make, can be mindful.

Recently, I noticed that when it comes to weight and weight loss, I have two types of students:

1. The students who maintain their weight and size yet grow stronger, happier and feel healthier. They feel more balanced in their life overall.

2. The students who slowly, gradually lose inches, drop sizes and fairly easily maintain their new lifestyle.

My students don't yo-yo. They don't lose weight dramatically only to regain it. As a teacher, I find this thrilling. No one is overly discouraged or distracted by feelings of "failure." Everyone lives life more empowered and positive.

I attribute this success to keeping the focus and priority on improved sensory awareness. Everyone is capable of tuning in and better interpreting messages from within their body. Therefore, everyone can achieve success!

Sensory awareness is the gift that keeps on giving. It constantly grows and increases in sensitivity. We continually learn what sensations we are seeking and what serve us positively. We turn inward and micro-adjust until we feel the experiences we are pursuing. A growth in sensory awareness leads students to feel more confident and comfortable in their own skin. They live life with greater inner knowledge and can't imagine their life any differently!

2. Improved Flexibility

An increase in flexibility is not measured by the ability to do the splits or touch one's toes. I don't remember not being able to do the splits. I consider the fact that I can still do them a very minor accomplishment. I am grateful for the flexibility but always confounded by the compliments. I have worked much harder at standing tall in Tadasana (Mountain pose) and relaxing during Savasana (Corpse pose) than I have ever worked at doing the splits.

There is natural flexibility that makes yoga poses more available and then there is flexibility that is earned. A positive change in flexibility is accomplished the same way tweaking is applied to food choices and strength training – slowly, steadily and consistently.

Dedicating time and attention to alignment in basic yoga postures on a consistent basis improves flexibility. Will the flexibility ever match what it was in our youth? Maybe no, maybe yes. It depends on what life has been lived between youth and present day.

Another question I often wonder – if we had actually been aware of proper alignment when we were kids, were we really as "flexible" as we remember? I watch the way children move all the time. I can tell you that most are hanging out in their joints – setting their bodies up to have the exact same aches and pains I witness later in more mature bodies. They just have additional cushioning inside their joints and are less aware of potential problems while participating in activities.

Have you spent the last few decades devoted to your flexibility and alignment? Or, have you been: chasing children, sitting at a desk or working on your feet all day? Entering a yoga practice with preconceived notions of what your flexibility "should" look like, due to imagined prior ability or a threshold of classes, only disappoints.

Instead, gauge how you feel post class versus pre class. Gauge what you can do after three months of regular attendance versus at the beginning. Basically, gauge whatever you can do today against how you were when you first started – this time around.

Do you remember all the facts that once helped you ace an 8th grade history test? Tsk, tsk, well why not?! Unless you are a history professor, history buff or have a photographic memory, why on earth would you remember every detail?

Your body works the same way. Just because you did something then, why would you now? That was then, this is now. You have filled your life and mind differently. You have different priorities today. Do you really want to relive the past? Embrace what your body allows you to do TODAY.

When we choose to shift our focus, then progress is viewed as PROGRESS. Improvement is exciting and uplifting. So **compliment yourself** on all that you can do today and **celebrate**!

3. Improved Balance – It's Loopy!

The ability to balance is linked to mental focus – which ebbs and flows throughout our day. Life is filled with distractions. Sometimes we can tune them out and other times we cannot.

The ability to balance is linked with physical organization, which requires awareness. Awareness requires sensing how to organize the body, which requires getting beyond the distractions within the mind.

The ability to balance is linked to self-confidence. Attempting balance positions can flood the brain with all sorts of negative thoughts and nervous anticipation. Merely uttering the word "balance" can throw us off, contributing to our cornucopia of mental distractions. Completely loopy!

Performance anxiety is a huge factor. When alone we can practice something *perfectly*, yet as soon as we're in front of others, we mess up. Are we suddenly less capable? Could we really have prepared more and experienced greater success?

- Balance is an exploration
- Balance is a practice for the mind as much as the body
- Balance is deliberate and mindful
- Balance rebels against hurry and expectation
- Balance requires practice; incrementally and steadily
- Balance requires positive, proactive self-talk

Olympic athletes practice endlessly. Their performance is just as affected by their state of mind (if not more so) as their physical readiness.

Recently, I added a balance station to my women-only circuit classes. It has been amazing to watch the transformation of attitudes and perspectives. The first week, I had the students simply stand on the flat side of the Bosu® ball. In anticipation, they all made negative comments about their "horrible balancing" ability. By the second round, they had to keep their mouths shut; otherwise they would have been total liars!

By week two, I upped the ante and made them stand on one foot. Week three, they were balancing on a single leg, hinged forward like an airplane. Each week, I increased the difficulty. I always have the Bosu placed near a wall for peace of mind. Everyone has to let go of the wall – even if it is just for a nanosecond. No exceptions! They are always able to balance far longer than they initially presume.

The students' improvements in balance and their shifting attitudes are some of the most gratifying and exciting experiences for me. And, I LOVE getting to say, "I TOLD YOU SO!!!" And ... I do a happy dance!

Balance improves with practice. There is always a loop, fending off distractions and self-doubt. But a positively shifting attitude assists and transforms the loop. Improved self-perception enhances our confidence. We are more adept at **allowing** ourselves to put a foot down, reset and try again. We know that we are capable. We understand that "balance is not a fixed state" in any part of our life. Needing to step off, prior to stepping back on, has absolutely no impact on our personal definition of how well we balance.

4. Improved Self-Confidence

We don't have to handle every experience we encounter with confidence in order to think of ourselves as confident. Yet, when it comes to our health and fitness, lack of self-confidence often spills over into other aspects of our life. We are held back and may not even be aware of it. Confidence in another area(s) does not tend to have the reciprocal effect. The fact that we have demonstrated an ability to learn, understand and even become good at "X" is not convincing evidence that we are equally capable of "succeeding" at our health and fitness. It is a perplexing reality for most women along their fitness journey.

In regards to fitness level, every woman has her own reasons for lack of self-confidence. It could be related to past "unsuccessful" experiences, other people's comments, etc. Every woman also has her own list of benefits when her confidence increases. Her reasons for lack of confidence or her list of benefits rarely has anything to do with the fitness activities themselves.

I do know that feeling more familiar, competent and confident at exercising and living healthy feeds into all other areas of our life. The reasons are endless and everyone would respond to the question uniquely. Maybe it is due to the release of endorphins or evidence of increased physical strength and ability, who knows? But I see it all the time.

Feeling more comfortable in any given situation boosts competence. Competence boosts chances and expectations for success. Feeling successful boosts confidence. Growing physically stronger, becoming more capable at working out, feeling more in charge of one's life and choices all boost self-confidence – an attractive quality creating its own very positive loop!

5. Improved Perception: Becoming a Snob ... about Form!

One of the hardest things I find about working out in public is that I have to put up blinders. Otherwise, I feel compelled to go around "helping" others with their alignment. It's an obnoxious quality and I work very hard to keep the urge in check. I see form first and ability second. A person's size and age are inconsequential to me but how a person moves in their body is either impressive or worrisome!

I find this quality growing in my students. I'm not sure if any would recognize it as a "success." But, I find it phenomenal. At one time, they would have been intimidated or discouraged by witnessing someone else's ability. They would have allowed the sight to interfere with their self-confidence. But as their knowledge level has increased, their insecurity has lessened.

Now, if my students look around at the gym or in class, it has no negative impact on their self-esteem. They know that form matters most. During my classes, I've had students give me a little wave and point to a fellow classmate because they were worried about their peer's form! Today, if they witness someone using poor alignment at the gym, they send a little prayer that the person doesn't get hurt! And, if they see someone using excellent form, they are duly impressed.

It's an amazing transformation. There is an absolute correlation between knowledge level and confidence. Knowledge IS power. Knowledge removes the power we previously relinquished to our imagined deficiencies. Anyone can work out effectively. Once the "how-to" is understood, comparison is moot. However, there is one hazard: you just might find yourself walking up to someone and offering unsolicited, possibly even unappreciated, but very helpful advice!!

Goals Shift With Time & Experience

Developing a consistent workout routine that is not loathsome is a big hurdle for many and a significant accomplishment! Once working out feels like a natural part of their lifestyle, clients **may** feel inspired to more actively tweak their eating patterns. The timing of this addition is different for everyone, from weeks to years. They feel so good from their workouts and suspect they could feel even better. They have more awareness of their food choices and are curious about doing things differently. They seek information about specific strategies. What I believe is integral to the successful process is that **the conversation is initiated by the**

client AND the impetus is positive. They feel good and want to feel better. There is no desperation, guilt or shoulds.

Still no overhaul, but we reassess their typical day and the foods that they love via the Health Map. (See the full version in the Resources chapter.) We discuss their motivations. I show them how to plan and tweak their current meals (one meal at a time). We brainstorm a list of items that can easily replace foods they are eating out of habit or convenience. We discuss mindful portions. We talk about the advantage of beginning meals with lean protein to feeling satisfied.

Slow and steady changes only. If they pin me down with a weight loss goal, then my response is 0, ¼ to ½ a pound lost weekly. Not fluctuating more than a few pounds during any given month is also an accomplishment.

****

A Word about Yo-Yo'ing:

I would rather a client's weight stay stable than yo-yo. The heart might be working harder at the heavier weight but it is accustomed to the load. A cycle of dramatic weight loss followed by regaining it is more stressful physically and emotionally. Not worth it and another advantage of tweaking!

****

Since working out is part of their regular routine, we discuss the concept of eating for energy. I ask them to notice their energy post-meals. No guilt – just awareness. What foods leave them feeling good? What foods leave them feeling overly full, drained or anxious? Choosing to eat something we know will be draining is not "bad." Nothing is forbidden. It is about choice. We **choose** the best "when" and "how much" to partake! We give ourselves permission to schedule the "treat meals." We consume with absolute joy!

Once clients are ready for empowered change, progress happens. Little by little, pounds come off, inches shed. A few months into the process they have demonstrable weight loss and looser clothing. Their strong musculature is more apparent and is always my favorite quality to point out!

Celebrate Success!!

Sticking with a workout regimen is an achievement! An increase in energy, strength and stamina are all successes. A couple months into our sessions, whether or not the body has visibly changed, I encourage clients to go shopping. I suggest they purchase a new exercise outfit or something (non-food) relating to their workouts.

If students experience weight loss and are swimming in their current clothing, they may be especially fearful to purchase new attire. I ask, "Are you struggling with your current lifestyle?" "Well, no." "Then, go shopping! Buy one new outfit or reward yourself in a non-food way, just do it." I am bossy – big surprise!

Wins must be acknowledged. We have to accustom ourselves, little by little, to our new and evolving identity – regardless of any so-called results. It is unsettling to view ourselves in new ways. Even when the changes are good, it is still scary. What if we fail? What if we make a fool of ourselves? On and on. Tell those thoughts to just shut up! They are not positive, purposeful or helpful! The mere fact of having those thoughts does not give them any credibility. They are just thoughts. **They only have as much power as we give them.**

We can't be afraid of our own successes and expect to stay on a positive track. We can't be afraid of our own successes and expect to have the strength – the courage – to deal with others' reactions to our new self. It takes time for others' perceptions to catch up. Having the tenacity to graciously handle other people's reactions during the adjustment period can feel taxing – even if everyone is supportive. We need to recognize within ourselves how far we've come in our attitude and our habits to fuel our confidence and self-belief. We need to invigorate and reinforce our positives so that we have the mettle to face whatever challenges – external and internal – come our way.

If we are not feeling bogged down by significant struggle – to be or continue on this new, healthier path – why would we backtrack? What would motivate us? Life is so good as it is right now, what would make us volitionally choose to regress to our former lifestyle? We won't. There have been no dramatic changes to the body, mind or soul to provoke rebellion.

We were inspired to change, not guilted into it. This healthier lifestyle has become a part of who we are – an improved version of ourselves – and we feel great. Vibrancy, happy mood and increased energy level are all signs of achievement to me. When I see clients coming to life, feeling better in their own skin, I feel my job is complete. That they continue on their healthful path is a given. I feel blessed to have been a witness and participant in their journey.

Even if/when clients' goals are achieved, most continue to take classes because they realize they are having fun and are grateful for the supportive community of like-minded individuals around them. Their surrounding peers notice their happier mood, stronger body and attractive, new clothing. The self-identified successful clients contribute to the group in new ways and motivate everyone else in their presence. It is a beautiful, exciting sight and completely contagious.

A Little Rant About Workout Clothing

Quit wearing your crappiest clothing to exercise! This is time for you to feel strong, empowered and motivated! What you wear affects your state of mind and attitude. Workout clothing should be wicking and feel like second skin. It needs to move with your body, not chafe or distract, AND, it should look attractive to your figure!!

Please believe me when I say, tighter clothing is more flattering. Wearing a too big T-shirt doesn't hide anything from anyone; it just makes you look bigger than you are. Tighter clothing might make you feel more vulnerable and self-conscious – I get that. Start out with darker colors. Find cuts that emphasize your strengths – and don't you dare say that you don't have any strengths! There is a right outfit for you. You will feel much better about yourself than when wearing ridiculously oversized T-shirts and raggedy pants. I promise.

If you feel attractive and invest some money on your exercise clothing, you will BE motivated TO work out as well as FEEL motivated DURING your workouts! Other women notice clothing – you will receive oodles of compliments!

You don't need to put on make-up or do anything special with your hair, blah, blah. But, you are NOT allowed to show up feeling that you don't even want to look at your reflection in the mirror!! How can that possibly be motivating?! You are worthy of looking sharp while exercising. You are worth the low-risk investment of a new clothing purchase, especially one that inspires dedication to this positive lifestyle. Pretty, pretty please?? **JUST DO IT!!**

Putting It All Together

Since deciding that I was in charge of the intention, my perspective of personal training has completely transformed. I've returned to it with a vengeance and love every minute of it. Students determine motivation but I dictate how success will be measured. And, I take great pleasure in pointing out my criteria very frequently!

I will not participate in any negative self-fulfilling prophecy. Students have to believe in themselves to spend time with me. I will drill it into them if I have to! I require them to say kind things about themselves, to measure their success from a different perspective and to appreciate aspects of themselves they habitually take for granted.

If they think negatively, they are not allowed to utter the words. If nothing else, it would not be good for the group. Everyone struggles with their own "shtuff," why on earth would we volitionally fuel the negative?

**We are strong and contribute to life in our own ways.
Thankfully, this is a journey filled with
lots of opportunities to practice!**

JAN SOKOLOFF HARNESS

58 years old
Married, two daughters

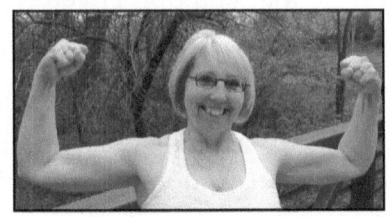

On the way to my first training class with Shanna, I stopped at a discount store and bought the cheapest yoga mat I could find. I'd been a yo-yo dieter and exerciser for years – I had no reason to think this go-round would be any different. I was wrong. I now consider exercise, yoga and mindful eating as much a part of my day-to-day life as brushing my teeth or saying my morning prayer. Dieting and exercising used to be something to accomplish and/or abandon. No more. Healthy living is now simply part of my life. My attitude has transformed, along with my perceptions of myself and other women.

I see myself differently and I see others differently

It's amazing to me when I look back at where I was a couple of years ago in terms of healthy living and where I am now. I probably wouldn't have started taking classes with Shanna, but things combined into a perfect storm. First, a client asked contractors to stop working on site, prompting me to work solely out of my home office. That was a real challenge, since my girls were both in school, my husband went to work, we didn't have a pet and the house felt very lonely. I needed some community.

The change in my schedule also gave me time to exercise – and that's no small thing. Going to a class at a set time every week isn't easy when you're expected at an office. So working at home, on no set schedule, made it easier for me to get to class.

The shape my body was taking also pushed me to go. I was no longer able to just jump out of bed in the morning and start moving, without aches and pains – the kind of aches and pains you hear about from old people. I was 55. I was not ready to feel old. Even more irritating was what I saw in the mirror. I was developing a dowager's hump, which is every bit as ugly as it sounds.

When I talked with Shanna about that, she very gently told me that she didn't know if we could reverse the damage done, but we could stop it from getting worse. I wasn't thrilled, but … I figured not getting worse was better than nothing. So, I put on my old spandex shorts and a 2X T-shirt and went to my first class.

Walking into that class was, in a word, horrible. The first person I saw was slim, young and beautiful. She looked like a ballerina. I didn't want to exercise next to a ballerina; I felt fat enough without that. Then, I got winded during the warm-up. Not good. Then, Shanna had us do some exercise lying down on a foam roller – those long tube things. I couldn't do it. I couldn't balance on the roller. I tried and tried and then I got really mad at myself for being such a loser. I gave up and walked out.

Fortunately, Shanna didn't make a big deal about it when I left – or after I regained my composure and walked back in. And the beautiful young woman proved to be truly beautiful: She gave me the warmest, most welcoming, understanding look when I came back in the room. It made me feel like there was hope, and that I really was somewhere I belonged.

And that's what's happened. Shanna, the other women – they've become my "peeps." With them as my community, I don't miss the office! Well, not as much.

Since that stressful first day, I have changed in remarkable ways. I hear Shanna's voice in my head continually, and it's a good thing. I pull my shoulders back as I walk, and I don't worry about good posture making my large chest look even larger. I stand straighter and taller – no small thing when you're as short as I am. I engage under my arms, not just in class, but when I'm doing housework or picking up groceries.

I was at the grocery store recently and the kid who was checking me out looked at me, looked at my reusable bag, and asked me if I wanted him to fill it up. I assured him that the bag was tough and so was I. Basically, "Fill it up, sonny." The woman in line behind me just laughed and laughed.

But the thing is, I am tough now. I am stronger than I have ever been. I've even improved my physical health. I was diagnosed with osteoporosis with a severe risk of fracture last year, and was placed on a medical treatment of a twice-yearly injection. I just went back for a second bone-density test, to see if there was any improvement. After one year, I have increased my bone density 8.1 percent. I had the doctor check to see how much of that was the meds and how much was my lifestyle. The average increase in bone density for a woman on the medicine I'm taking is 3.2 percent. The doctor was really excited and proud of me and I'm proud of me too. The exercise and eating right is paying off.

This is a huge thing for me. I've almost moved the osteoporosis measurement from "severe risk of fracture" to osteopenia – a condition far less serious. I've watched my mother get old and fragile and break. I know what that future looks like, and while I'd like to get old and still be as feisty as she is, I don't want to be as fragile.

I jump out of bed ready for the day to begin – no aches. No pains. The dowager's hump is almost gone. Not completely, but no one would notice it. I actually look at myself in the mirror now and love what I see. I stand in front of the mirror and make muscles. That may sound really goofy, but it makes me feel good to see how strong my arms and shoulders are, and how straight I stand. I still prefer loose shirts when I'm out and about, but I wear fitted exercise clothes to work out in. And I'm starting to feel more comfortable in regular clothes that really fit.

I see myself differently and I see others differently. I don't judge myself by the number on the scale – which hasn't moved over the past two years of exercise, even though I've lost one or two dress sizes. And I don't judge other women just because they're a size 4.

After two years of healthy living, I feel like a new and improved me. And that makes me really excited for the future! If I'm strong now, just imagine what I'll be like when I'm 65!

VIII. SEVEN POTENTIAL FACTORS OF WEIGHT LOSS

1. Adaptation

At some point, every student will come to me and say that they are easily maintaining but not losing weight. I ask how they are feeling in terms of energy level, mood and overall quality of life. I explain that this might be the weight their body needs to maintain for a while or indefinitely. Can they live with that? Typically, the response is yeeesss – maybe not the happiest "yes" but life is good and yo-yo'ing is not appealing.

The most significant improvements to strength, endurance and weight loss occur when the mind-body connection connects! This might happen early into the process. It can also occur after several years. The point being that when sensory awareness feels most dramatic within, external results will also be at their most dramatic. Then, the body adapts and expects maintenance of the status quo. It has become used to current activity level and calories consumed. Improvement can still take place but it will be less dramatic. If we want different results, we have to do more and eat even less – or differently.

As of this moment, I teach 14 classes/sessions weekly. Additionally, I walk 45'ish minutes most days and take classes up to 6 times weekly. I'm guessing that I eat around 1800 calories daily. Many people would expect me to be able to eat whatever I desire. If I do, I will gain weight. My body expects my level of activity, quantity of calories and type of calories. If I go off the map, my body rebels.

The body adapts. The journey is FOREVER. You have to find the equilibrium in your lifestyle that makes your body AND soul happy. The specifics of what that looks like are different for every individual and evolve with time.

2. Extremes!

Just like our mind and emotions, our body enjoys the status quo. If you have ever quickly dropped a significant amount of weight, only to even more quickly regain it, ask yourself: did your body seem to participate in the self-sabotage via intense cravings, plateaus, fatigue and irritability? Like a little devil was sitting on your shoulder – offering endless temptations and daring you every step of the way?

The body is not okay with extreme measures. It is not going to accept them. The body will rebel. Then, the mind and emotions will feel defeated, resentful and give up on the process.

For most of us, sustainable improvements occur by:

1. Avoiding extreme measures (in either direction)
2. Requiring the focus to be on positive results of: energy, endurance, stamina, strength and any others named by you!

Focusing on the positive ... striving for balance ... greatly minimizes the opportunity for self-sabotage on all levels.

3. Food (of course)

As much as I love working out and teaching fitness, exercise does not guarantee or necessarily even lead to weight loss. Exercise will make you stronger, your heart healthier and present tone when weight comes off. But for weight loss, it's mostly about the food intake. What we eat is at least 80% of the equation – my personal guesstimate.

Everyone knows individuals who are slim and don't exercise at all. They just know the right portions for their body's needs. That doesn't guarantee they have strong bones, muscles or a healthy heart.

Exercise makes you pretty on the inside. I liken it to someone who only brushes their teeth but doesn't floss. Your teeth might be pretty and without cavities but your gums are going to drop those teeth way sooner than someone who is flossing!

4. Comparisons!

No one else has your exact same personality, life experience, values, memories, physical body and so much more. You are unique and have your own body shape and strengths. Respect and celebrate what your body allows you to do. I assure you, there are things you can do that someone else skinnier, stronger, younger or more flexible cannot do. There is always a hidden talent taken for granted.

On a physical level, someone's hamstrings are more flexible but their hips are tight. Someone can do heavy bicep curls but can't figure out how to engage their back muscles. Sitting, someone can easily touch their toes when the legs are together but as soon as their legs are extended out to the sides, they can hardly sit up straight.

I watch it occur all around me in classes and hope that students are noticing their strengths. Of course, they barely seem to acknowledge or notice … until the person next to them can do something "better." Then, they wonder, why can't they do it too? Do we recognize the 2-year-old within?

Our bones are put together in a unique way. We're similar enough that we are all in the human family, but there are endless, subtle differences that impact our strengths and challenges. We each live in our own body and are used to its abilities and talents. So, we don't notice.

Of course, I have to embarrass students. I make a point to show an unappreciated skill they do with ease – they have no idea how it could be challenging for anyone else in the room, yet it is. I love to watch the shift in their expression. A recognition and appreciation for their body's abilities moves in, rather than solely focusing on what they lack. Mission to redirect – successful!

We are Unique! Duh!!

I used to work at a high-end athletic clothing store. I interacted with women at their most vulnerable. They were self-conscious about skin protruding – no matter the area. The bra area, middle section, butt, thighs, the side back – otherwise known as "back fat," on and on … you name it, they mentioned it – negatively.

It was a surreal experience. I constantly wished that all the women could see and hear one another. What one woman perceived as negative, another would kill to have that problem. At one point, I realized that I was doing the same when trying on clothes; looking only for the so-called "problems." I had more skin hanging out around the front and back of my bra than when I was younger. My middle wasn't as tight as it used to be. Cellulite was more noticeable, on and on.

Now if I do that, I just tell myself to shut up! I would not dream of thinking, let alone uttering, those words to any other human being. Why do I dare say them to myself?

Line up 100 women who weigh the same number on the scale, we will see many different body types, shapes, heights, breast sizes, waist sizes, musculature and softness. Additionally, a 32B woman will not have the same overall size as a 32DD, 38C, 36A, etc. Bra size is part of the proportion of a woman's body. Even if two women are the same height and approximately the same waist size, their weight on the scale will be different. All those body types lose (or gain) weight and tone completely differently.

There is a difference between wanting to feel attractive in our own skin versus holding ourselves to an unrealistic (or even impossible) ideal. If we are alive, then we have skin, muscles, bones and fat. We get older and gravity has its effects. We are not supposed to look or be "perfect" – ever!

Early on, we learn to hold ourselves to an unrealistic ideal. Did we even appreciate the vigor and energy of our youth? Most likely not. We took it for granted. Are we making that same mistake now? In 20 years, will we look back on images of our younger bodies/selves and mourn what we still did not appreciate?

Many of us attempt to be everything to everyone. We attempt to be perfect physically … perfect managers of our time and energy … perfect in our every role with every significant person in our life. Physical perfection is not possible. Perfection on any level is not possible, and moreover it is ill advised. In the mere attempt to look or be perfect, we lose our individuality – potentially disappointing ourselves and everyone else. Let's try our best and accept, laugh and ask forgiveness for what goes awry along the way!

Real life is humbling. Messing up, being imperfect, provides the potential to learn more and do better. Imperfections and quirks make us relatable and approachable. Is there anything more obnoxious than people who seem to think they are perfect?

Let's be **positive** examples of real'ness and empower others to do the same!

5. Fatigue and Lack of Energy

As I write this, winter is in full throttle. This morning it was snowing and dark. It was the quintessential morning to sleep in. In order to get my tired butt out of bed before 6 a.m., I had to visualize my day (based on a great deal of previous experience) with two possible scenarios:

1) If I slept in
   a) I would have the immediate reward of extra sleep
   b) The remainder of the morning with the kids would be rushed and stressful
   c) I would feel behind throughout the day

d) I would re-remember that the extra 30-60 minutes of sleep did not provide a noticeable increase in overall energy ... AT ... ALL

e) I would end the day feeling mildly dissatisfied for once again "failing" myself and the effect that it had on those around me

f) I would wake up the next morning with all the same dilemmas

2) If I got up

a) I would have immediate awareness of fatigue

b) My shower would need to occur instantly in order to truly wake up – and I still might need coffee

c) My morning with the family would feel a bit sleepy but not rushed

d) I would have time to get a lot done prior to teaching my morning classes – i.e., take my morning walk, make two days worth of salads, write, get in a load of laundry, etc.

e) I would be on time or ahead of the game for the rest of the day

f) I could easily justify taking a 30-minute nap prior to picking the kids up from school or before teaching my evening classes

g) I would get to the end of the day feeling a certain level of pride in the fact that I got my tired self out of bed by the designated time

h) I might feel a little more motivated to get myself into bed at an earlier time of night!

i) Maintaining a positive pattern, regardless of temptation, would make getting up by 6 a.m. tomorrow just a tad easier

Most of the time, I choose option two. The temptation to sleep-in always exists, but it doesn't typically win. Prior evidence is stacked against it. Exceptions are made for illness and snow days or other extenuating circumstances. But, through a lot of trial and error, I have found life to be far more pleasant and successful if I just get myself out of bed – on time. It is a prime example of delayed gratification offering greater reward.

Creating positive habits takes effort and is rarely easy. A big part of me would LOVE to sleep in – especially in the winter. Nine months of the year, I am dedicated to my morning 5K. I feel on top of the world and unstoppable. Then the winter hits – along with my humility. I surrender to the treadmill (or not) and inner negotiations.

At first, I still get three'ish miles accomplished but gradually my distance goes down to one mile AND I am proud to have endured! Sheesh. I can't wait for "Spring Shanna" to return! Then the cycle begins anew. "Winter Shanna" endures … sometimes just barely. "Spring, Summer and Fall Shanna" are happy, happy, happy and mostly remember to be grateful!

Energy – Can I Have Some More Please???

Is there a magical formula to increase one's energy? It seems to be the modern day alchemy. So-called energy boosts are displayed and advertised everywhere – none will be promoted here. I'll leave that to others.

Barring any medical issue that could be impacting your energy level, my belief is that you've got to spend some to get some. I typically do not feel more energized by lying in bed and watching television all day. I just feel depressed and unaccomplished. I do feel more energized post working out. My mind feels sharper and I am proud of my efforts.

I allow and look forward to rest and relaxation every evening and weekend. I view that as part of maintaining a positive life balance. But R&R don't feel fully deserved if I haven't done something to earn them. I pay the mortgage before I purchase new clothes. I eat the healthy stuff before the sweet treat. I do my "Have To's" before my "Want To's." It just makes sense to me and I have significant evidence in my life that it is the better strategy.

I think most of us are wishing for more and more energy. We watch children in wonder. Did we really feel like that once? So, we negotiate, we cope, we manage, we practice, we try over and over again. We work to build the personal evidence, inner drive, that makes choosing better feel easier. With that evidence, we strive to have the energy to get what matters most to us accomplished AND feel fabulous about our efforts. Like everything else, it is a practice.

6. The Scale

The scale can be used as a tool, as one measure – but not as THE measure. It can be used as a checkpoint once in a while but not as an obsession. I weigh myself weekly at most. It is always in the morning, without clothes, before eating and after doing my business!

Today at 40 years old, I weigh 15 pounds more than I did 20 years ago, but my waist size is pretty much the same. Do I love seeing the heavier weight? Eh, it is not my favorite thing. But, I can't and won't focus on that. How would getting stuck on a number serve me well? I have energy and vitality. I have strength and far more self-confidence than I did at 20. Hallelujah!

I enjoy how I look with and without clothing. I think my shoulders are terrific and powerful. I don't want to return to being 20, so I'll accept the number and move on. It is only one number and doesn't tell my full story.

I weigh myself to stay aware and keep myself in check especially during times with greater temptation. I also understand that my weight fluctuates three'ish pounds every month – no matter what I do and it always has. So I don't get hung up on it.

Physically, my weight doesn't communicate how many straight leg push-ups I can do, the strength of my abs or that I can shake my booty in Zumba® class. How does your weight not tell your full story? What does it not say about you? What physical, mental and emotional strengths does it not measure? What are your talents? If you choose to use the scale as a tool, how can it be a positive example to others around you?

Most people would not guess that I weigh 120 pounds: they often think I barely weigh 100. I gladly share the number. If it benefits anyone, then yay! I don't pull in my belly or hold my breath for any picture. I will not go on a special diet for a photo shoot.

I live my life, eat what I love and participate in activities that feed me on all levels. We are constantly modeling to others. If we complain about weighing a certain number, what is that communicating to other souls in our presence? How does uttering those words or using that kind of language positively serve our environment?

The scale is **one** tool – don't let a number steal your thunder, enthusiasm or energy in any way. You are WAY more than that. Do you hear the homophone? You are **WAY** more than you weigh!

7. Holidays and Festivities

Holidays seem endless. Thankfully, there are oodles of reasons to celebrate: special days, birthdays, and on and on. Food is always central. My goal for the holidays is to enjoy myself in a balanced way. I think it is unrealistic to go into Thanksgiving, for example, and expect to lose weight. I strive to keep it all in check and enjoyable.

This Thanksgiving let's be in a better place (mentally, physically and emotionally) than the previous Thanksgiving. Every year we know more about ourselves and, therefore, can enter each holiday, each celebration, at an even better threshold.

The "Strategies" section has specific ideas regarding how to enter all holidays and exceptional days. Most importantly: setting realistic expectations, having kind thoughts toward yourself and repeating compassionate words over and over again!

Factors – So What? How Much Do They Matter … Really?

There are valid factors to weight loss. Some are within our control and some are not. We can approach the seven factors (or any else that we know about) with knowledge and awareness. We can **manage** our factors. Ultimately, they can't be our daily focus. They aren't motivating. Most importantly, we can't allow them to be **demotivating**. We can't allow our factors to rob us of incentive and enthusiasm for living a healthier lifestyle.

Truth is truth and facts are facts. And, so what? Truly, who cares? I am listing them in this book as acknowledgement of a reality that exists for most of us. Do not surrender your power to whatever are your factors. They are a part of our lives but they don't have to rule our lives unless we accept that mindset. Any factors of weight loss should not impede you from enjoying your life – right now. They should not discourage you from choosing more positive options.

Factors exist in any challenging scenario. It is the process of overcoming and persevering that is motivating and inspiring – regardless of the obstacle. See and believe in your strengths. Honor authentic measures of success mentioned in the previous chapter. Reflect on how much more you understand about yourself today in comparison to what you knew yesterday. Allow that to serve as evidence and promise of all that still remains to learn and discover about yourself in the years to come! Be excited! You are alive and have the power to set the tone of your life. Factors are called *factors* not *motivators* for a reason. **Factors** are aspects, issues or features. **Motivators** are instigators, cheerleaders and inspirations.

Know and understand your factors. FEED your motivators!

IX. LEARNING & GRIPPING

One of my most frequent teaching cues is *relax the tongue*. We habitually grip our tongue to the roof of our mouth as though that action will assist our focus and ability. Typically, we are totally unaware that we are doing it. Sometimes students will ask how I know – because I always seem to know. Here's the truth: yes, I can tell because the back of their necks look stiff or their faces are tense; but often I know because I just noticed that mine is gripping too.

Gripping is like white knuckling. The hand might be able to hold on to an object but circulation is being stunted. At some point, the hand will go numb and drop whatever it is holding. Gripping, holding on for dear life, is an emergency move. It is not an action meant to sustain us long-term. Gripping should come with a warning – we are not breathing or at least we are not breathing smoothly, deeply and calmly. Gripping the tongue sends messages throughout the body to grip and clench.

Does trying to balance on one foot qualify as an emergency? Do most decisions or attempts warrant that kind of tension? I feel like I am speaking to myself because I am a quick gripper. It is only in yoga and exercise when the noise leaves my mind. I experience inner quiet and perspective. I am utterly calm and centered.

Otherwise, my insides are humming. I have to move my body to quiet my easily anxious mind. I have learned techniques that help me feel grounded and mindful. In the busy'ness of life and all my many roles, exercise makes me feel sane and I am so grateful for it.

Learning: Practicing the Attitude of a Practicer

Just because I practice and teach yoga does not mean I am immune to stress. Just because I work out and eat healthy doesn't mean I am invincible from illness or cravings. Just because someone is an "expert" doesn't make them infallible. We are all practicers at all aspects of life. Some areas are just easier for us to practice than others.

Being "all grown up" does not mean that anything should come easily or that we will instantly be good at it. We still need patience, determination, a sense of humor and willingness to practice – over and over again.

Learning: Phases of Learning – A Cumulative Effect

Learning something new can feel overwhelming, especially as an adult. Many of us are accustomed to being experts in our field. Being brand new to a subject is humbling. We need to be interested enough in the topic to accept the difficulties of the process.

Learning a new subject requires learning a new language. Every topic has its own lingo. And every teacher uses her or his own shorthand. I try to warn all my new students that learning occurs in phases. Relating to exercise, it goes something like this:

Phase 1: *"Huh? My foot goes where? Wait a minute, say what?"*
My heart always aches for new students because it is
OVERWHELMING. I always tell them that I know they'll hardly
hear most of my cues. I understand where they are at and explain
that it is all going to be okay. Phase One mostly involves gross
motor skills, the figuring out of what goes where. In Phase One,
we feel sluggish, clumsy and disorganized.

As soon as we get everything positioned "right," the body moves
– seemingly of its own accord and without our awareness. It feels
like we never progress beyond square one. We feel inept and
dumb. Please give yourself a break AND a ton of compliments for
giving it all a chance! The good news? Phase One is the shortest
phase. Hallelujah!!!

Phase 2: *"My muscle does what?"* Now that the feet are where
they are supposed to be (and mostly staying in place) and the
bones are facing the right directions, it is time to figure out how to
engage the muscles appropriately and effectively. This phase
takes a while because we have muscles that easily engage and
others that have been sleeping for quite some time. The real fun
and organizing begin in Phase Two. With practice, we become
more efficient at firing everything in unison – no matter the
position. But, this is a process and what makes the topic so
interesting. If it were easy, would we really stick with it?

Phase 3: *"How is my breath moving through my body?"* Phase
Three lasts forever. It is all about the subtleties. It is where the
magic happens. Throughout any exercise or yoga pose, attention
turns inward to the pattern of our breath. We tweak. We micro-
adjust until our body feels the most benefit in each position. With
every breath, we explore our edge. Phase Three is introspective

and meditative. Phase Three is being "in the zone." It is the bomb. **I LOVE and relish Phase Three!**

Starting out, learning a new subject, we can't jump to Phase Three. That's an anomaly if it occurs. Skipping the earlier phases of learning wouldn't be fair to all those individuals who've dedicated time and energy to the subject. Therefore, the optimal benefits from any exercise regimen do not occur right at first. I know it kind of sucks but it also kind of doesn't. Phase Three is the reward for effort and focus. It is earned. As we move through the phases, our questions grow in complexity. The results are more satisfying and juicy.

If you don't loathe an exercise then allow time to explore it. Allow your body and mind the chance to learn how to communicate with one another. Over time, you will more efficiently organize and "get it." It's impossible to judge by taking one class. The brain can't even process the majority of information to relay to the body!

I know that most of what I say goes over people's heads at first. I expect it and am tremendously grateful when students return! I love it when I hear comments like, "Shanna, today in class, you said <cue X> and it was so helpful. You really should say it more often." I always express gratitude. It doesn't matter that I have been saying that exact same cue during every class for months or years. The brain hears what it hears when it is ready to hear it and not a moment sooner. I celebrate the fact that their brain and body heard the information!

Take baby steps. One of my favorite aspects of parenting was having the opportunity to relearn subjects with my children. Greek mythology or Shakespeare written for kids is so accessible!!

It makes returning to the "grown up" versions far easier and satisfying. Expect the phases of learning, celebrate your ever-growing ease. It's a chance to enjoy the benefits of childhood without all the other crap!

Gripping: Brain Interference

The very first time I took a golf lesson, my initial swing was beautiful and the ball went straight and far. I didn't even know I could hit the ball! My instructor said I was a natural. Then I thought, "Oh, %$&! I've got to do that again? How did I just do that?" Of course, on the second attempt I swung at air.

My brain got in the way. If my body had been left to its own accord and my mind remained quiet – without expectation – I probably would have at least hit the dang ball. My mind interfered and I gave credibility to the fear, expectation and uncertainty.

We often buy into our misperception and over generalization and then we let it lead us. A big part of my job as a yoga/Pilates/whatever instructor is to get beyond the student's self-limiting thoughts. I am trying to assist the student's mind-body connection and bypass self-judgment.

Gripping: Just Because We Can – Doesn't Mean We Should

At the same time, I am trying to impart that just because we were able to touch our toes once upon a time does not mean it will – or even should – happen today or a year from now. A lot of life has been lived between then and now! Unless there's been continuous practice of those specific moves, why on earth would our body easily go into them?

In a yoga class, we are just regular peeps, practicing something that is **supposed** to decrease our stress, make us feel stronger, taller, more limber and balanced overall. We are not competing with anyone around us or some former, imagined version of ourselves or what we "used" to do … back in high school or college? 30 years ago? BK (before kids)? Pullease. Let's give ourselves a break.

I have been practicing yoga daily since 1999. In my youth, I was a student of ballet, tap and jazz. There is a lot of momentum behind my abilities. And, there is no need for me to be stupid just because I used to do a certain pose early in my practice. My life, body, priorities, values are all different today. What exactly is my intention? Am I trying to prove something to myself, show off or feel better in my own skin?

Learning: Practicing Appropriate Effort

Sometimes 70% effort is enough and what is most appropriate. If it has been a long time since your body has done certain moves, then don't make your first attempts "all guns blazing." Your body won't approve or acquiesce safely.

The body responds to tweaking on all levels. So, no big overhaul allowed when it comes to exercising. Let go of your ego and pick up the three-pound weights or whatever qualifies as light. You are not being wimpy … you are being smart. And who cares what absolute strangers you may never see again think of you? They don't know you and most likely they aren't even looking at you!

No matter the exercise, the body is carrying its own weight, which after many repetitions of the same movement can be tiring. Many repetitions can also challenge physical alignment. As our body tires, we tend to focus on getting through the moves rather than remaining aware. We might not even know our body's response to the exercises until 72 hours later.

Until and unless excellent form is learned, the risk for injury is high – no matter the lightness of weight or number of repetitions. As our body ages, it is less forgiving of improper form. There is less cushioning in our joints. The after effects are more obvious than when we were 20. The creaks and stiffness, the fatigue and soreness are all magnified and less tolerable.

I can feel it in my own body and I've been consistently exercising for years. I cannot put forth the same intensity and determination of my 20s without a greater physical cost. I am highly motivated to have excellent form because the smallest misalignment creates far more irritation than it ever would have 20 years ago. I don't want to lose time in my life to pain that is avoidable.

The good news is that I am smarter today than I was then. I don't want to go back to any previous age. The benefits of my life today far outweigh the costs of not being able to do the exact same things in the exact same ways as my past. I am willing to pay more attention as well as take less for granted.

Learning: Conscious Exploration

Conscious exploration is finding the balance between what was and what is. Habit can lead to assumptions. Often, we are completely unaware of our limiting assumptions. We find ourselves stopping at a certain depth in a yoga pose or a number of repetitions when lifting weights merely because that has always been our limit. "That's all I can do. This is where my body goes, it doesn't go further because that's all I've ever done." Self-limiting assumptions do not take into account the momentum of practice. We are always growing, learning and evolving.

Without judgment or expectation, approach any movement with "I wonder if ..." It is all just an exploration. Most of the time we surprise ourselves. A yoga position or exercise is only as stagnant as we allow it to be. The edge constantly moves. The movement might be infinitesimal! No one needs to experience the inner growth other than you! The visibility of your progress will show up in other ways, i.e., standing taller, feeling stronger, etc. Exploration is part of the journey of learning.

Learning: Community

As stated in Chapter 5, a learning community of like-minded peers can be vital to motivation and success in learning. Your right community has nothing to do with your size, age, ability or income. It has to do with finding peers who have similar interests and attitudes. With these people you feel at home, they bring out the best in you. Having your right learners around you feeds your motivation, self-belief and ability. It is invaluable.

Who is your right teacher? This is another exploration. He/she tends to draw your like-minded peers, so looking for them can lead you to the right individual(s). I love to look around my classes. The students are so varied from age, size, experience, career and background. But I swear that I have one student – because their essence is so similar. They would have a great time if attending the same party. My students laugh, encourage one another, have huge hearts, give each other and myself a hard time and hold each other accountable to get to class. In a word, they are – magnificent!

Learning: Rules of Engagement for Exercising!

When it comes to learning how to exercise, let go of expectation for "the burn," heavy sweat or exercise high. Instead, focus on:

1. Quality over quantity! One repetition completed with excellent form beats a plethora of those performed with poor quality – no matter the calories burned. Poorly performed repetitions will be ineffective at best or lead to injury at worst.

2. Tweaking strikes again! Strive for incremental challenges to strength and endurance. Test the edge of your strength and endurance by slowly increasing the amount of weight lifted, the number of reps performed or the depth in a yoga pose. Learn how your body responds to the increased effort during your workout as well as 72 hours later.

Safely testing the threshold for quantity of repetitions leads to an increase in stamina and endurance. Safely testing the threshold for amount of weight lifted leads to increase in strength. There is no reason to rush this process! There are big reasons to broach cautiously: you want to be able to walk, wash your hair and live your life without feeling paralyzed by soreness!

3. Happy joints! It is vital to listen to your body. Increased strength, stamina and endurance will ultimately happen but not long-term if at the expense of your joints. Harm to any joint is a major issue and sometimes a permanent setback. Be patient with the process and release expectation of results. Having happy joints is vital to living well in your body. Honor where your body is today. Tomorrow may be a totally different scenario – let's make it one for the better!

Gripping: No Hunching! Slouching is Forbidden!

I have yet to witness a sport where the athlete is taught and encouraged to hunch.

A hunched position is some combination of the following:

- Upper spine is rounded outward
- Shoulders are elevated and forward
- Chest cavity is dipped inward
- Low back is either overly rounded outward (while seated) or overly dipping inward (while standing)
- Head of the thigh bones are challenging the groins by protruding forward (while standing) or upward (while seated)
- Center of the knees are not centered between the center of the hips and ankles
- Weight is unevenly distributed within each foot and between the two feet

Mindlessly hunching occurs constantly … at the computer, in the car, standing in line, walking, talking, doing, being … ALL – THE – TIME.

Some possible physical effects of hunching:

- Breathing is shallower since the breath doesn't easily flow to the low belly. This can lead to increased tension mentally, emotionally and physically – especially around the lower back and/or neck
- Upper back muscles are over stretched from the frequent slouched position. This can make those muscles weaker while providing less sensory input

- o Weak upper back muscles increase stress on the neck and shoulders. This can cause the neck muscles to feel tight which can lead to excessive sensory input which can then lead to frequent clenching of the jaw, tongue and throat
- Joints are challenged because they are habitually misaligned
- Joints and low back are "clogged" due to blood not flowing around them or through them efficiently, potentially leading to stiffness, soreness and/or swelling
- Ankles, feet and other areas of the body are stressed due to carrying weight unevenly

Physically, hunching makes the body heavier on the joints. It makes some muscles overstretch and weaken, leading to decreased sensory input. Other muscles overly grip and tighten – leading to sensory overload and tension.

A muscle is only as strong as it can engage. If a muscle is constantly gripping (engaging), it won't be able to grip much more – if at all. Can a light be turned on more if it is already turned on? Maybe, if it has a dimmer switch. Accessible strength from overly tight or weak muscles are either dimmed or turned off completely.

Emotionally, hunching feels heavy, stressful and down. Hunching creates a defeatist mindset. On the opposite end of the spectrum, when we are angry, we stand taller, cross our arms to protect our heart, or use our hands to strongly express our point. The defensive stance is stronger and more powerful but overly tense and stressed.

Either extreme is not beneficial. We don't want to live with a defeated or survivalist mindset. We want to live empowered and mindfully aware.

If hunching causes so many problems, then why are we habitual hunchers?

1. It is easier in the moment
2. It does not require a great deal of awareness
3. It does not have obvious or immediate consequences

The consequences of hunching build over time. At the point our body is in trouble, it becomes difficult to recognize the relationship between our sufferings and our habits.

How we move is a telling map for our habits. I'll often ask a new student if they have any prior injuries of which I should be aware. The typical response is, "No, not really." Then we start moving and suddenly all kinds of aches and pains are "remembered." Those aches and pains are just not thought of as injuries. Now, I am realizing that I should rephrase my typical question!! My new question will now be, "Do you have any regular aches and pains of which I should be aware?"

Learning: Never Too Late to Make a Shift

It really is never too late to make a shift in your life and your habits. You don't know the future. No matter your age, you still might have decades left, how do you want them to feel, to be?

My parents were in their early 50s when they decided to start a band AND be DJs. My sister and I were both mortified and inspired. We went to some of their gigs. It felt completely weird and required a paradigm shift. My kids thought it was cool and my then 5-year-old daughter loved getting on stage with them. My 20-something sister, who lived at home at the time, had the pleasure of asking our parents to please keep the noise level at 1 a.m. to a minimum because she had to work the next day!

It was awesome, funny and gave me a new perspective on aging and trying new things. It is in the not doing everything perfectly that spices up our lives. It is in the trying new things, laughing at ourselves and trying again that we discover new aspects of ourselves and others.

I have endless, encouraging and funny stories of my family. They were not led by fear when it came to trying whatever they thought was interesting. They didn't care what others thought. Anyone who judged them had no business participating in their lives. Trying new things made them feel more alive and youthful. They always surprised people with their brand of fearlessness.

Those memories inspire me today.

What is it you want for yourself? What do you dream of trying if not held back by fear of failing, looking foolish or feeling disappointed in your current abilities?

Your entry point to living a healthier lifestyle is yours to discover and explore. Make a list of all the activities that sound even remotely appealing. Pick up a catalog, research online for ideas. Try a Groupon™, LivingSocial™ or some other deal to sample. Talk to individuals you enjoy being around or admire. What kind of activities do they enjoy? A gym membership is a possibility but not a requirement to being active. I love taking classes. I have found different studios that I love. Would you prefer to take walks on your own or would you like a buddy?

We are constantly modeling to those around us. What would you like to inspire in others? Be it your children or a complete stranger – you never know the effect you have on those around you. Let's be compassionate learners, try'ers and practicers. Who knows where it all can lead?

ANNE SCHULTZ
67 years old
Married, four daughters,
seven grandchildren

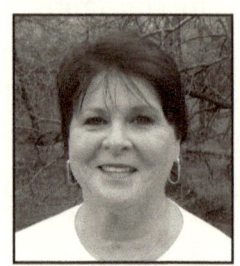

One morning, before Shanna's circuit training class started, Anne Schultz mentioned that she and her husband were planning a big family vacation to celebrate their 50th wedding anniversary. All of us in the class thought we had misunderstood. When did Anne get married? When she was a toddler? Turns out, we heard right. Anne married at 17; she and her husband celebrated their golden anniversary on a trip with their children and grandchildren. Today, at 67, Anne is an inspirational example of how healthy living can help a woman maintain strength, energy and an amazing youthful glow.

Exercise makes you feel good. So go! Work out! What have you got to lose?

Healthy aging is taking care of yourself physically, mentally and spiritually. When you do that for yourself, it makes your whole life fuller.

I married at 17 and had kids boom, boom, boom. I'm glad I did; now I'm enjoying my grandchildren. My kids and grandkids keep me young – I've gotta be on my toes for them! Our whole family is always active.

I have exercised on and off since my 40s, so I've been taking classes for over 25 years. My goal now is to just firm up and be more agile. I don't want to be one of those people who can't get off the toilet without the help of the countertop. And I know the more you exercise, the less health problems you have. I hit 60 and started thinking about these things. I know it's good for me – it's a great benefit for longevity.

Since I started exercising years ago, I've been in many classes and been to many gyms – and I never met anyone like Shanna. I wish we had met 10 years ago! She is the only person that I can remember who called before my first class and talked to me. I was so surprised; I even remember where I was! I was at my daughter's house and I answered my cell phone. It was Shanna and she wanted to know all about me.

No one, all those years, had done that. Now, I've been working out with her for over a year. When I travel for pleasure and work, I miss her classes. But I hear Shanna's voice in my head. "Stand up straight! Shoulders back!" Or, "Imagine you're on the foam roller!"

I don't eat like Shanna, but I'm more conscious now in making food choices and how I look at labels. One of my daughters put me on that path. We're lucky to be in a time of life where there's so much more research on food and the chemicals that go into food. And I do listen when Shanna talks about food. She's walking energy, so when she tells me what's good, I believe it! And I'm trying to eat more fish.

I made some salmon recently, sprayed the pan, put the fish seasoning on, baked it for 10 minutes and it was awesome. Eating better really takes less time – making lasagna versus salmon in the oven? It's a no brainer. And the more you eat certain things, the more you get used to the taste. There are just two of us in the house, so we typically have a salad, a piece of fish or meat and some veggies.

I am trying to lose 10 pounds, but it gets harder as you get older. I've given up certain things and I still don't see a change of weight. One time I eliminated alcohol for Lent and I didn't lose a pound. Shanna says, "Don't be so conscious of your weight – it's more how you feel inside." She's right, but I know what shows on the outside too!

I had a breast reduction years ago and I'm glad I did – it was one of the best things I've ever done. I was a 40D and the bra straps were always cutting into me. It wasn't cosmetic. It was more about health. The surgery made me feel so much better. All the weight I was carrying was dragging me down.

I do think I've aged well. A lot of people my age are out of shape and having health problems – some are even dying. But exercise makes you feel good. So go! Work out! You know it's good for the insides of your body to get your heart going. I say, you don't have to start with a vigorous workout. Start with 15 minutes and work your way up. What have you got to lose?

I took a boxing class recently. My grandson needed someone to try it out so he could get in a drawing. He's in high school. His dad, my son-in-law, and I went. They wrap your hands, put on gloves, the whole bit. We did 15 minutes on the bag and the rest of the hour was running, calisthenics, jumping jacks, lunges. Every time the instructor would say, "Get down and do pushups," we went down and did pushups. My son-in-law kept coming over saying, "Are you OK? Are you OK?" I made it through the class just fine and at the end my grandson said, "Dad, Nani did better than you!"

X. STRATEGIES

This is my least favorite subject to discuss or write about because people's tastes are so varied and personal. Since the idea is to sustain a healthy lifestyle, I don't want to insert a feeling of obligation or guilt. Take all these strategies as suggestions. Give a whirl to those that appeal and discard the rest. Whatever you choose has to work for YOU, your lifestyle, your tastes – period.

I am neither a nutritionist nor a dietician. These strategies are based on my continual learning as a fitness instructor, life experience and anecdotal evidence. Nutrition and fitness advice are like any other science; the information evolves, ebbs and flows as new data and awareness come to the forefront.

A while back, people were afraid to eat avocados due to fat content. Today, we know the difference between healthy and non-healthy kinds of fats. We are still learning. Judge your success based on how you feel physically, mentally and emotionally. You are the only one who has to live your life.

My son has Crohn's. He cannot eat what I eat. His body absorbs nutrients differently. What I eat would create additional inflammation within him and lead to a flare up. What he eats would make me lethargic and balloon. The family is in awe of Aaron's diet – his meals seem endless. Where does it all go? He is a skinny weed. But he is growing and thriving, so we accept that his dietary needs are different and try not to be jealous!

It seems like we all know people who thrive on eating whatever they want. They are the exception, which is why they stand out in our mind. Like people who have an endless income and can buy whatever they desire – those individuals are rare. So, ask yourself: in this moment, for this meal, what would make me feel successful?

Quantity, Quality and the Order of Things

For me, the answer is to start with the good stuff and make the majority of the meal "good stuff." Half my dinner plate is veggies, one-fourth or so is lean protein and the remaining is typically something like quinoa. My theory is … if I fill up on the healthy, there is less space for the non-healthy or less healthy, i.e. dark chocolate covered almonds.

Typically, I eat the protein first because it is most filling. I proceed with the veggies and then end with the other carbs. If I am still hungry, I will enjoy extra veggies and protein. I rarely eat much in the way of pasta, bread or anything in that family, regardless if it is whole grain or not, because it drains me of energy and makes me feel bloated. I eat enough to quench the craving for the texture and flavor. Depending on the food, I season with herbs, vinegars, and sometimes olive oil or coconut butter.

When I am almost full, I eat a small dessert. And, chewing gum is very comforting and satisfying. Sometimes, I go a bit overboard with the gum! I don't chew for long but I love chewing multiple pieces simultaneously. It's just so juicy! It protects me from overeating. I chew long enough for my brain to receive messages that I am actually full and there is no room left for additional food.

Cravings – Negotiating like a Pro

When my belly feels like a bottomless pit and I am facing serious cravings for sweets, I typically start with fruit. I still get my chocolate, I just don't start with it. When I am craving salty, I go for veggies, nuts, and then the chips and salsa. I self-negotiate so there is less room for the treats. I don't want to start with the stuff that would feed my guilt or steal my energy. I negotiate, so that I can feel proud of myself for keeping the craving manageable. I win!

I use the same strategy before heading to a party or a festive meal; I eat something healthy and energizing before I leave, so I am not arriving hungry. I am not without temptation. I work to minimize its power.

Cravings are a part of life. Just because we start or are living a healthier lifestyle does not mean we are cured from, or are immune to, temptation. The key is to find methods to deal with those cravings and still live happily within your body and mind.

Enjoying vs. Gorging

In my not-so-distant past, I LOVED frosting. In my childhood, it was all about Cap'n Crunch's® Crunch Berries® cereal. There are foods you love and have a healthy relationship with and foods you LOVE and have zero self control. For me, the latter does not enter the house.

I still blow kisses and feel a little angst every time I walk by Crunch Berries at the grocery store, but I know it cannot come into my home. If you do not feel in control and will be living with regret, then it just seems mean to have the item(s) in the house. It also sets you up for feelings of failure.

I have absolutely no self-control or ability to negotiate when it comes to those foods. I can easily eat three or four large bowls of Crunch Berries. I can and have eaten an entire top of a sheet cake (all the frosting plus a little bit of cake), YUM!!!

I LOVE the flavor. I LOATHE the effects. It is awful. First, my belly hurts which creates its own source of panic. More than my bellyache is the emotional roller coaster.

It all starts out fun. Initially, I am flying HIGH. I find everything hysterical, especially myself. I laugh and laugh. Unfortunately, the happy phase lasts no more than an hour.

I spend the next several hours, SAD, really sad, like my whole world is just so sad. I feel bad about myself and the burden I am to others.

When the sadness dissipates, I get MAD and pissed off at everything. When everything in the world irritates you, it is a clear sign the problem is not the world, the problem is YOU.

This entire process takes at least 24 hours to clear, sometimes longer depending on the quantity of sugar consumed. The "pissed off" phase lasts longest, probably because that is where my personality most easily goes. Stress on the system just exacerbates whatever exists within us. Fun times!

A "Support" Network

My husband, children and sister all have to experience these phases right along with me. So, they tend to monitor my food choices very closely at any celebration. They also retell stories from the past just in case anyone in attendance doesn't know or remember.

It then seems like everyone is on watch to see if or how much cake I consume. I used to sneak into the kitchen and steal spoonfuls of leftover frosting. I thought I was so clever but I would always get the giggles. Needless to say, I have pretty much earned those watchful eyes – so I don't resent them.

I didn't set out to have this kind of "support" system but I know it comes from love and not wanting to have a total bee-yotch in the house.

We benefit from having different kinds of support systems in our lives. This particular example saves me from seeing the worst of myself come to fruition. I don't feel mocked or defensive, I feel supported and accepted. I know my family loves me no matter what and they are really just looking out for me. We are a "teasing" kind of family and if anyone crosses a line, we have absolutely no problem communicating it!

Dynamics in families and friendships vary. Individual needs vary. My example might be your worst nightmare. If that is the case, don't establish or accept anything like it. If you choose to create a support system, then ensure it is YOUR definition of supportive.

No Deprivation!

On the flip side, denying yourself foods you love equally sets you up for failure. The only time in my life I have ever thought much about food was when I thought I needed to diet. I was in college and had gained a few pounds. All of a sudden, I was thinking about food ALL – THE – TIME. I was thinking about my next meal and how many cookies I was allowed. It was horrible and it hardly lasted.

I loathed what was happening to my mind and emotions. Who was this person inside of me? That was not me! I decided that I was just going to do my best and not allow myself to be obsessed with food nor every single bite I consumed.

At some level, I understood that I was going to make mindful choices. If I was going to obsess – then let it be things I have always obsessed about – why on earth would I willingly take on something new??!!

So, no deprivation is allowed. If I feel like having dessert, then I have dessert – at a serving size that feels appropriate and satisfying. I consume it with awareness and pleasure. I really enjoy those dark chocolate covered almonds but I can't eat them straight out of the container as I can mindlessly eat twice the serving size. I split the serving size into two mini baggies and that is my quota for the day – well, at least, most of the time!

Handling a Host(ess)

I can empathize with someone who spends a great deal of energy, time and possibly money on entertaining, only to have any guest(s) consume very little. It would feel totally offensive. For the sake of full disclosure, I think everyone has given up on me. So, I do not feel much pressure to partake, no matter the event. I also have strategies.

For the following reasons, I am always the first in line for food:

1. It gives everyone else permission to get in line. I have never understood why so many people are shy about being first in line for food, but I am happy to ease any discomfort.

2. I, the germaphobe, get to be the first to touch everything. Less hands = less fear. I can't tell you how many times I have said, "You touch it, you take it!" And I was not speaking to children.

3. I get the most options possible. I load my plate with veggies, vinaigrette salads, lean'ish protein and go light on anything else. However, my plate looks full. I walk around with my full plate for all to see and position myself so that many people can see me eating. This way, I can say and be believed that I already ate, it was wonderfully delicious and I am happily full.

4. I place what looks like a reasonable amount of items made especially for me on my plate. They are usually dairy-free but still have too much sugar, fat, etc. Sometimes I taste it, sometimes I mess around with it on my plate so it looks like I ate it. Child's tricks still can work as adults! And, sometimes I eat the whole amount and enjoy it. Whatever I eat is with full awareness.

5. If alcohol is being served, I will nurse one glass of wine the entire time. I am not much of a drinker but this one action seems to put others around me at ease. I don't mind the taste, I don't want a refill and the heat is soothing. So, I just carry it around and take small sips when conversing with

others. Another option is to get sparkling water with lime – no one but you will know the difference.

Making Compromises

I feel guilty writing/thinking this, but most of the time, I really wish no one would go to the trouble of making food especially for me. I don't give it the love it deserves. It just isn't my currency. There are **special** foods at **special** times of the year that are **special** to eat but not at every single celebration/get-together otherwise how on earth are they **special**?? It is too much. Too, too much – for me.

We all make compromises in the company of others. None of us acts the exact same way around others as we do when we are alone. When encountering a food dilemma, use a strategy that serves you best and that you can most happily live with – in each scenario. Personally, I think lying about the quantity you eat for the sake of a host's happiness is permissible. If that is how they express love, they may never understand how you could refuse.

You have to gauge it by the relationship. My grandmother never understood and always resented my "lack of appetite." I really could have and should have lied (at least a little) for her sake.

With my dad, there was no way I would have gotten away with lying. We worked at finding common ground so that he wasn't constantly irritated with me. He finally asked me what would I eat? I told him what I really, truly loved. So, at get-togethers he made authentically healthy options – exclusively for me. I was beyond grateful and relieved. I made sure to always arrive hungry. To this day, sautéed mushrooms remind me of my father. He didn't even use oil. That, my friend, is love.

Eating Out

1. Full disclosure and hardly shocking: I rarely eat out. It is rough out there in restaurant world. EVERYTHING seems to be high in sodium – even if it is "healthy." Most things are really high in calories, saturated fat, etc. Unless you are going to a restaurant that lists every ingredient and all the nutritional facts, it is very easy to underestimate what you are eating.

2. If I've been invited to meet up at a specific restaurant, I try to investigate the menu and nutritional facts online ahead of time (if they are available) and have a plan on what to order – combined with eating something ahead of time at home.

3. I take dessert with me in my purse. It sounds like a crazy old lady taking food home in a napkin – in reverse! I want and love dessert. Restaurant desserts are LOADED (and they typically have dairy anyway). So, I bring something sweet with me – in a controlled portion that I can eat and feel satisfied. People who know me are used to my antics and tease me – but I am okay with all of it.

It is plain and simple; I want to feel good **ALL** of the time. I want to spend my life and my time well. I want to spend quality time with all the special people in my life.

Teaching yoga/Pilates/strength training when you feel gassy, bloated, lethargic or have heartburn is NOT FUN! It is not a casual discomfort, it completely sucks … been there, done that.

I teach five days a week. I am highly motivated to eat with awareness and be at my best for my students and for myself. On the weekends, I still want to feel excellent because that is time with my family. I do not want to waste time in my life – in bed or on the toilet – from self-induced reasons. Eating particular foods or quantities, that I know don't serve me well, wastes my time and my energy.

I have learned the hard way that because I eat a fairly clean diet, my body and mood are very sensitive to going "off the map." What causes major suffering for me is minor for everyone else in my family. When I first realized this truth, I resented the fact that I actually **had** to maintain my lifestyle in order to consistently feel good. Feeling at my best most days wasn't accidental! Then, I decided that resenting the truth was more draining than motivating. I chose this lifestyle. No one imposed it on me.

Forewarning: the more you choose what feels best for you, the more your life might actually REQUIRE it! But, it's all good because the reward far outweighs the cost.

Peer Pressure (Real or Imagined)

Since the time my daughter was a very little girl, we've had conversations about body image and healthy living. I knew that once she was fully grown, there was a high likelihood that I would be smaller than her. We have different body types and food preferences. I was VERY worried about how that would impact her self-image. It is not the typical order of things. Most moms are bigger than their daughters. I didn't want my lifestyle to harm her in any way.

On the flip side, no matter the love, I wasn't willing to sacrifice my entire way of being to potentially make her feel better about herself. So, from a very young age, I taught her that we create our own definition of happiness. I told her that what made me happiest and feeling at my best was eating a lot of fruits and vegetables and exercising. But, it is not how everyone defines happiness. Mackenzie quickly agreed that it was not how she would define happiness.

I explained that my lifestyle kept my body at a certain size. When she got older and her body finished growing, she would most likely be bigger than me. I explained about our different body types and how we liked different foods. At five, Mackenzie said that was perfectly fine because she was not about to eat the way I ate or exercise as much as me.

Great – I had set the groundwork.

Puberty hit and it still wasn't easy. No matter how much logic and awareness exists, puberty is rough and imposes tons of change. So Mackenzie and I continued to have heart-to-hearts. She wasn't mad at me, but she acknowledged that life would feel easier if I wasn't so damn small. (Mackenzie wants it known that "damn" is my addition!)

Today, Mackenzie is happy and confident in her own skin. She makes mindful choices and owns her life. I've given her the techniques, the rest is up to her and she is good with that.

Feeling Responsible for Others or Vice Versa

Most of us have someone(s) in our life for whom we feel responsible. We want to make them feel more comfortable with whatever their choices are and, in turn, have them feel comfortable with our own. It is tempting to change or do things "for them" that you wouldn't otherwise choose.

Or, maybe it is you who craves permission when making certain choices. The idea that if you are "treating" yourself, the treat tastes even more delicious if someone else is eating it right along with you or encouraging you. Well … and there is no nice way of saying this … it is simply not fair or right.

You want the treat? Have the treat! But don't rope someone else into it so that you can justify it. It still has all the same calories.

You want to eat healthier? Great! But, don't obligate everyone around you to make the same choices just because you are now ready.

The topic of food is sensitive enough without imposing obligation in any direction. No one should be guilted or pressed into eating something healthy and equally so when it is not healthy. We don't want anyone to sabotage or put a stumbling block on our personal journey. The same is true for how we treat others.

We all have to find our own balance, our own path

Thankfully, we possess and get to express free will, which means we are responsible no matter what. What mom hasn't told her kid, "I don't care what (insert name) was doing. You made the choice right along with (insert name) and you have to deal with the consequences!"

We get to be the navigator of our own life. For most situations, we cannot authentically say, "He/she made me do it." We made a choice. We chose to say "yes," we chose to give in, because it was easier in the moment than being completely honest. Fine, but we own it. We allowed ourselves to feel obligated. So be it – but it was still a choice.

I could have put the pressure on myself, felt obligated to my daughter (whether or not it was what she truly wanted or needed). I could have made some aspects of my family's life easier in the moment by giving in and saying yes, but at what personal cost – on so many levels?

We need to be our authentic selves – especially with our loved ones. I could have lied to Baba once in a while about whatever quantity I had or had not consumed, but I could never have lied all the time – and she never would have wanted me to … not really.

No one is a threat to your path unless you allow it. You are not a threat to anyone else's path unless you impose. So MYOB* and others will too … at least most of the time.

*MYOB = mind your own business! Check Chapter 13 for further details.

Cost/Benefit Analysis: Is it worth it?

Is that particular food worth whatever the known aftereffect is? Are the taste, calories, etc., worth it? Only you can answer that question for yourself. Mindful choices, being responsible for yourself – that's being a grown-up. So, pause and ask yourself, is it worth it?

If your answer is yes, then enjoy! Every – Single – Bite!!!

If your answer is no, step away. Just – Step – Away.

These days it really is not hard for me to have a little piece of cake or none at all at any celebration (with or without witnesses). The personal price is too dang high. I love and am very grateful for my life. I don't want to volitionally screw it up, not even for 24 hours. It is not how I define "living."

A cost/benefit analysis is my constant method of choice – no matter the currency. *Making mindful choices is the easiest path to living life with few to no regrets. Doesn't that sound delicious?*

Forgiveness – You Never "BLOW IT" so Get Over Yourself!

So, you binged. Who cares? That doesn't guarantee or warrant a reason to binge some more. You are not a failure. Take a deep breath, assess the situation that preceded the event. What's done is done. Reassessment is not about judgment or guilt. It is about learning how to protect yourself in the future and setting yourself up for success.

Did you bring the "gorging foods" into the house? Did you use some stressful event as an excuse? Are there other strategies or distractions that you can implement in the future to better handle whatever was the trigger, such as going out with friends, taking a walk, heading to the library?

Gorge – Guilt Free!

I love the library as a strategy. Can you think of a better place to gorge? Everything is FREE! Zero cost, zero calories and LOADED with information. I LOVE libraries, museums and parks. Raising kids on a tight budget meant I learned a lot about how to entertain them for free or with very little money.

Not only were those places cheap financially but they also passed the time in a positive, productive way – a very important technique for a stressed-out parent with small children!

We all have a 2-year-old living inside of us who wants to be entertained and comforted. We need to be our own parent. We all have our go-to strategies.

Replace, retrain and redirect in other ways you find pleasant ...
and take a healthy snack with you!

The key is to have a plan ahead of time. Make a list of all the places and activities that you enjoy that never lead to a sense of regret. What feeds you – mind, body AND soul? Food does not have a monopoly on our happiness and life satisfaction.

I gorge on books, DVDs, CDs from the library. I go to the bookstores and look at EVERYTHING that interests me. I love used bookstores! I love art. I love looking at ETSY.com. Walking outside is my lifeline. I love listening to music – the familiar and exploring anything new. The phone! Talking to loved ones who "get you" is priceless. These are only some of my go-to strategies for dealing with stress, boredom or loneliness. I feast my eyes, ears and mind – taste is not our only sense worth feeding.

Finding your methods is part of the journey of learning about and living with yourself. No judgment. Explore! You are more than any one thing.

As far as anyone knows for sure,
we are given this one body,
with this one mind,
in this one life.
What do you really want to do with it all ...
each moment ...
of every day?

What Limits??!!

Are you really going to let yourself be limited by anyone else's definition of ... whatever it is you are allowing limit you? You really can do just about anything if it is worth it to you. Are you interested enough to make it happen? Sometimes, the answer is no. Sometimes, the answer is not yet. And, sometimes the answer is please, please, YES!

When I started teaching yoga, I was scared. I mean SCARED! I talked to myself aloud as I drove home after every class. I told myself, it was all going to be okay. I would only get better with practice and the only way to practice was to keep doing it.

I planned out my classes, taught to invisible people, taught my little children, made flashcards with cues, talked to myself in the mirror, wrote out transcripts, on and on. I practiced in every way I could imagine.

I went to tons of workshops, studied book after book after book. It didn't matter that I had had years of experience with my personal practice AND had already completed a teacher training. It didn't matter how much I knew in my mind. Teaching real live people (especially adults) is its own huge endeavor entirely.

All I knew for sure was that it was worth all the anxiety, self-doubt, fear and hard work. I knew that from the very first class I taught – where someone actually stormed out of the class, obviously displeased with my teaching style as the substitute teacher. I was so hurt and yet, I had to keep going. I had to get through it. The 60 minutes was agonizing. I wanted to cry and run away from the humiliation – but that was not an appropriate option.

Beginnings are rarely easy or smooth. It is not called beginner's luck for nothing – if it works well at the start, that's lucky but the easy phase doesn't last long. At some point, anything successful requires work, practice and many humbling experiences.

Making it Successful

Success is not typically accidental. We are driven or motivated to make things successful. I worked really hard and continue to work hard to feel successful at teaching. The only difference between teaching fitness, and any other previously attempted occupation, is that it was and is worth all the effort. It doesn't even feel like "work." I've worked harder at it than any other job outside of parenting. It's worth the sacrifice of time, money and energy. It was worth it. It is still worth it.

Working at something you love leaves you feeling inspired and elevated. You can't wait to do more of it. Working at something you don't enjoy leaves you drained and tired. You find all kinds of excuses to avoid or delay the work.

If you are truly motivated to make a change in your life …
If you feel positive about the effort …
If you practice regularly …

Then without a doubt, you will be successful. It is the bonafide truth. Is it immediate? Do most of us win the lottery? No. Immediate, positive results are not the definition of success. If so, I would have called myself a failure after teaching my very first yoga class. What a sad, sad story that would be for me.

I found something worthy within myself to keep trying … to put myself out there, in front of others, over and over again. It was painful, it was trying, there were wins and many setbacks. I kept plugging away. Today, there is nowhere I feel more at home and confident than teaching adults how to exercise safely.

I know my students are in knowledgeable and capable hands. I feel good about my teaching methods. Does this mean I am perfect? Am I done learning? Hardly! I learn from my students' questions and perspectives and tweak my methods daily.

I learn and I adjust. I mess up and I grow. Is every class stellar? Not a chance, but I keep at it. I give it my best effort. I don't define myself by my mistakes. I am my best efforts. I am doing the best I can with what I know in this moment … and so are you.

In college, I started out as a business major. Within three semesters, I was on academic probation. Business was definitely not my passion. I changed majors and all of a sudden, studying was interesting and I started getting As. Just because I was not good at business classes did not make me dumb, it just meant I was on the wrong path. But, I could have given up on myself and said college was not for me.

So, get back on that horse or whatever has knocked you down – try a different strategy. Try a cow or a duck! Try and try again. Something, at some point, is going to stick and prove successful … it will. It really, really, really, really will.

I can put endless "reallys" in front of "will" but it won't matter unless you make that promise to yourself and actually …

BELIEVE IT!

XI. HEALTHY LIVING AS A "FOREVER-TERM" INVESTMENT

Life can feel like a total crapshoot. It's kind of shocking how much in life seems to require a leap of faith. I remember being fully aware of this when the kids were little. I had no idea if my strategies and philosophy were going to produce good kids – the ultimate goal for any parent. I was guessing constantly and just doing my best. At times, it was petrifying!

Today, I have more confidence. The kids are by no means "all done," but there is more evidence in my methods today than when they were two, and they seem to be turning out well enough! I'm still guessing but the learning curve is not as steep.

The same goes with my health. My intention, as long as I'm alive, is to live well. My hope is to live a good, long life. I have no idea if what I'm doing will really make any difference 20, 30, 40 years from now. I hope it does, but I have no real idea, no foolproof guarantee.

What seems to be true is that the choices I'm making today are having a positive effect on my life – today. That the choices I've made until today have served me well. For the most part, I feel good physically, mentally and emotionally. I have the energy and drive to do the things that matter most to me. I feel satisfied and engaged by life; therefore, I am motivated to keep on with my experiment.

Based on evidence, I am willing to make the "Forever-Term" investment

~ but it is still a leap of faith.

We take leaps of faith all the time. We make purchases and have general performance expectations based on previous experience and evidence of the norm – but there is no actual guarantee that all will go smoothly.

We buy a car and strongly suspect that if we never wash it, never change the oil, never take care of the ongoing maintenance, then at some point – and we have no idea when – it will break down and get all rusty.

We could also do everything according to provided recommendations and it may still break down … early into the purchase. But, if that situation occurs, we get angry and demand a refund or some sort of recompense. Our experience did not fit expectations, so we take action. We pursue a different result.

That's not exactly an option with our body – there is no one to ask for a refund or demand recompense if it breaks down. We have to deal, manage and cope. We can pursue "repair" via medicine and treatment, but we are still the ones experiencing all the effects and side effects.

Our body doesn't come with a guarantee or an exact owner's manual. So, we pursue maintenance via trial and error and leaps of faith.

Responsibility: You Touch It - You Take It

In order to deal with the stress of unpredictability, I try to focus on what I can control. One of my personal lessons and what I teach my kids repeatedly: I don't want to purchase anything that I am not willing to maintain. The idea that "we touch it, we take it." We purchase it, we are responsible for it. We **agree** to the purchase, we are **still responsible** for it … for better or worse.

How we take care of it is our choice, but it still **belongs** to us. Overall, the quality of its life is in our hands, inanimate or alive. Our home (or room), yard, appliances, pets, body and on and on are ours to manage.

Before purchasing anything, I ask if it is worth the known maintenance costs in time, expense and energy. Are we willing to do the work? If we are unwilling to do the maintenance, is it replaceable and can we afford the additional expense? This process can be tedious but often far easier than dealing with the reality of an "unexpected" crisis or family drama of pointing blame.

In a way, I think of the body as a continual long-term investment that I **choose** to purchase (or repurchase) and maintain daily to the best of my ability and awareness. I don't always enjoy the maintenance but overall it seems worthwhile to sustain my quality of life. I don't always want to brush my teeth or wash my face at the end of the day when I am tired. I also don't want cavities or acne!

We all make purchases. Some items we enjoy so much that we name the maintenance of said purchase a "hobby." We work on it for countless hours but would never term it as work because we gain so much pleasure from it. Finding ways to maintain our body with the same mindset as a "hobby" can help us stay the course long-term.

The Journey is Forever

We own our body for our entire life. We have no idea if we will acquire a serious illness or get into a life-altering accident. It is important to plan and prepare for the exceptions as best we can, but most of the time, we are hoping to live well on a day-to-day basis. We might assume that tomorrow (and many tomorrows following) will be pretty similar to today – or we are working very hard today to make our tomorrows even better – or maybe we have given up entirely.

I don't want to live from a place of deprivation nor desperation. I want to feel at peace with all my decisions from the mundane to the significant. I try to make mindful choices for the best experience possible – in the here and now, immediate future and potentially long-term. I want to be able to look at myself, at the mirror within, and say:

"You're doing the best you can with what you know and you are doing well. Keep learning and you'll keep improving."

Consistent Truths

When I teach yoga and fitness, I strive to give consistent cues no matter the exercise and no matter the body's relation to gravity. What is true in every pose? What can be reaffirmed in every position? Many, many, many, many things (see an incomplete list in the "Resources" section). I try to give consistent messages so that the students can more easily integrate the information.

On occasion, there are exceptions and I explain the reasoning behind those exceptions. Explaining the intention for exceptions quiets the perplexed mind. Explanations bring a sense of inner peace and acceptance.

But, overall, for the students to feel independently successful and organized, they cannot memorize unique qualities in every pose. Overall body organization and alignment cannot constantly be situational or how would anyone ever learn how to do anything? Based on prior experience and evidence, we should be able to infer and extrapolate as new situations arise.

Our brain seeks consistencies in all aspects of life. Our brain seeks explanations to exceptions. Truths with a capital "T" are universal, no matter the subject. Those "Truths" can be applied to any concept and any job in any field. What is always True for you?

Some of my Guiding Principles:

- Mindful living is more effortful in the moment but far easier in the long run than being reactionary
- Practicing mindful living becomes more habitual and less effortful over time
- I work best with a plan of action
- I prefer to assess all dilemmas with a cost/benefit analysis
- I strive for balance, no matter the currency
- Currency – time, money, calories, energy – requires all the same methods for success. I choose to complete my "have to's" before pursuing my "want to's"

- I value security, safety, healthy longevity and inner wisdom so those values guide my choices
- I am my best teacher and trust my inner voice. I strive to pay attention to internal warnings
- Reminders (warnings) whether they come from within or an external source are gifts – heed them
- I strive to try my best, reassess and forgive
- If I keep my focus on the bigger picture (the higher purpose) then the necessary details become clearer
- It is always helpful to take a smooth, deep breath
- I have to feel purposeful and passionate about my life
- I shouldn't do anything FOR long-term results that I'm not willing to DO long term
- I should speak to myself in the same ways I would chat with my best friend; honestly and respectfully (not defeatist or rude)
- I'm allowed to change my mind as long as I understand my intention
- I'm not supposed to be perfect at anything but I am supposed to keep practicing – I am a practicer

I think articulating what is always true for you is an invaluable exercise. Where in your life do you feel in charge? Why is that? What are the qualities that make you feel empowered? What are the underlying principles that guide you in that area of your life?

Where and why do things go awry elsewhere? Are those "off" areas significant enough that you are motivated to make lasting change?

Not every aspect of our life requires the exact same kind of attention or effort. We have to find our own style and allow ourselves permission to shift and change along with our priorities.

I love consistency, regardless of my role – wife, mother, fitness instructor, synagogue volunteer or driver on the road. I want to feel in charge of my life and have found ways to make my bossiness work for me. And, hopefully, for those around me!

We all have strengths regardless if those strengths are recognized by others or ourselves. Analyze what makes you feel confident and competent at (fill in the blank) and find the themes that can be applied elsewhere. Those skills are already a part of you, they are your gifts to be harnessed, in any area.

Real Truths with a capital "T" are beautiful and empowering. When I understand something about a yoga pose that could be said about any aspect of life, it feels like getting a peek into the bigger mystery of LIFE.

Those statements, those truths, are everywhere and in everything. I could read a book about improving my golf game and apply all the underlying principles to eating healthy, pursuing a degree, going for a bike ride, etc.

Tap into your strengths. What do you know 100% about yourself? What absolute consistencies do you recognize about life? For everything else, what, within you, are you willing to invest in on a "forever-term" basis? Are you willing to take a leap of faith that your efforts, your commitment, YOU are worth all the work, time and energy? I hope your answer is *YES!*

MACKENZIE HAUN
16 years old
Single

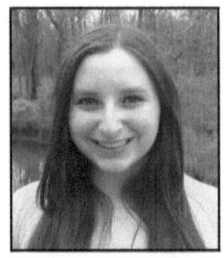

Picture your mother in your mind. Does she look like a lithe, lean yoga machine? Now, consider this: would you want her to? How would you feel if your mother was visibly smaller than you are? At 16, Mackenzie Haun readily accepts that she doesn't look like her mother Shanna – and never will, no matter what eating plan she follows or how much she exercises. Mackenzie and Shanna have very different body types and personalities. Does it matter? Not anymore. A teenager wise beyond her years, Mackenzie realizes how she and her mom differ and, more importantly, what they share: a desire to live healthy, be happy and help others.

I don't feel the way I felt before any more. I feel strong.
My mom never did this and I'm glad, but I have friends who feel pressured by their moms to be smaller. If I could tell mothers something it would be, "Don't do that. Believe me, your daughters know how they look and they know how they feel." I don't know anyone who hasn't gone through some sort of self-esteem issue as a teenager. Help them find ways to feel better about themselves. They may already look great – but that won't matter until they feel it.

I spent a semester in Israel this year and went through a real transition. There was a group of 21 of us and we got to see most of Israel. I was in the IDF (Israel Defense Forces) for a week. I went to Poland. I walked from Galilee to the Mediterranean. We went to Masada. I was climbing mountains fairly often, walking everywhere and eating differently. Even without really trying, I trimmed down.

We were taking lots of photos, so I could see my progress on Facebook. But the real change – it's not so much a visible change. It's a change within me. I really gained self-confidence and felt so different when I returned – like I was not the same person, but in a good way. The experience was really good for me in terms of confidence. I don't feel the way I felt before any more. I feel strong.

Before I left, I was not in a very happy place. I was just a down person. I didn't have a very positive attitude about anything. That had an impact on what I ate – I just didn't have a conscious approach to eating. I was working out once in a while, but not every week, and I wasn't motivated. I wasn't mindful about eating or exercising.

Now that I'm back, I want to be active and make better eating choices. I enjoy the benefit of it. My mood is improved and I feel better. Living healthy to me is eating what I enjoy but being conscious of what I'm eating and how it affects my life. I exercise three times a week – I do cardio once or twice a week, Zumba and weights.

When I'm doing weights, I'll go on the machine after someone who looks really strong and then I can lift the same or more! And I just think, "Ha! I may not look strong, but I am." And sometimes people are lifting more, but in bad form. And I'm doing it in the right form so I don't get hurt.

I don't think I look scrawny, but I don't have the typical look for a strong person. I don't do sports. I'm not ripped. But it's all a matter of perception.

Strong can't be defined by how you look – especially for women. We don't bulk up easily. My mom is really strong, but it's much easier for Dad to bulk up visible muscles. If I were defining *strong* as a feeling, it's just something you have to find within yourself. You can't get it from a list of conditions. There's no formula for feeling strong – I wish I had a formula. I wish I could say, "This is what you need," but I can't. It just has to come from within. It's not magical. A weight isn't going to make you magically happy. You'll get to that weight and find something else is wrong. Your physical shape can't define your happiness.

But being physically strong and emotionally strong do go together. My mom says it all the time: "Don't diet. Just live your definition of a healthy lifestyle." Mom always tells me, "You will feel better after working out." It's the endorphins, sure, but it's more than that. If you feel like you can do something you didn't think you could do, that makes you feel stronger in the rest of your life. I can give you two examples. When I started sophomore chemistry, I had a C and I didn't think I'd get over a B. When I went into the final, my grade was over 100, and that felt amazing!

Also, I had – and still have – a severe fear of heights. It was crippling. I would shake. In Israel, the first mountain we were going to climb was Masada. It was not a good day. We were climbing at 4:30 in the morning and I was tired and didn't feel well. When we got to the top of the mountain, a couple of us were given the option to take the cable car down. But I chose to climb, and that was the hardest part because I was so afraid.

When I got to the bottom, I thought, "I just climbed a mountain!" I felt so accomplished! My friends were so proud of me and I was so proud of myself. I probably shouldn't say it this way, but I felt like a bad-ass! It was such a great feeling.

Now that I'm back, I can see how much I've changed. And I don't mind putting my story out there if it will help others. If I have a message, it's this: "Try to get to a place where you feel good about yourself."

XII. CONTINUAL METAMORPHOSIS

One morning, out of the blue it seemed, my dad woke me up at 7 a.m. on a Saturday to go running. I was taken aback but amenable. Running didn't seem all that exciting but being the firstborn, I never wanted to disappoint Dad. He seemed so excited, so pumped up. I think I was six or seven years old (all I know for sure is that it was before I was in ballet classes).

This was the first of many Saturday morning runs with my dad. They were a blend of running, walking, lecturing, tears, laughter and closeness. Many Saturdays, we would run-walk-run to McDonald's™ where we ate breakfast and then woke Mom to come get us. I don't remember ever making the return trip home – much to Mom's chagrin!

It was only a few miles (three at most) but it felt like a major accomplishment. At the time, Dad said that he initiated it because he was worried I was becoming lazy. Truly, I think he was restless and bored and I was a willing partner!

Some Saturdays, we would go to the high school track. I'll never forget the one day he told me to spread my arms like wings, close my eyes and feel the magic of the wind – like flying. It was fabulous and after a moment I told him so – only to hear someone else's voice tell me that was wonderful... but that he was not my dad. Startled, I opened my eyes to see my dad far ahead of me doubled over in laughter.

It was hard to actually be angry or maintain mortification because it was so funny. I still gave him a hard punch on his arm (our expression of love) but we both cracked up throughout the rest of the run and every time we returned to the track. He was always doing "shtuff" like that and I was almost always falling for it. To this day when I think about it, I have a blend of disbelief that he would do such a thing and another voice that says, "of course he would!"

Prima Ballerina

I was always dancing around the house. I can't remember which came first – the leotard or the classes. Some people sing in the shower, I danced in the shower. I danced when brushing my teeth. I danced without knowing that I was dancing – all this is still true today. So, dance lessons seemed completely natural.

The classes fit my appreciation of structure and made me feel accomplished. I loved the repetition, the practice and all the new ideas. I loved the clothing, the community and the independence. I loved the challenge and feelings of success. I had something that was all my own.

One day after my scheduled class, I was watching the next one. The front desk ladies told me to just go in and take the class. I wasn't sure if I was allowed but they insisted. At the peak of my lessons, my parents would drop me off after school and pick me up around 9 p.m. a couple times a week plus occasional performances. The experience was thrilling.

After a while though, it was also stressful. As I grew older and improved in skill, the pressure to be even more serious increased. Ultimately, my family was worried about the financial cost of lessons as well as the cost to my peace of mind. I was starting to get stressed about the littlest things. My parents were trying to figure out if I could dance casually. Did I want to switch to a different studio with a more flexible philosophy? I couldn't figure it out. One day, right before junior high, my parents ended my dance lessons. All of a sudden, a major part of my identity had disappeared.

An Early Identity Shift

I felt somewhat lost but also relieved. I loved dancing but not enough to pursue it exclusively or with such seriousness. I think I was curious about what else life had to offer outside of dance.

From junior high through my early twenties, I wasn't active in any kind of structured way. I still danced in my room, took walks, went for family bike rides, did a little Jazzercize®, but I did not think of myself as athletic. When I look at photos or videos during that time, I can see that I am skinny soft and it showed in my personality.

My father had an ongoing frustration in my lack of direction or self-confidence. It confounded him, but I never could identify the reason or how to change it. He wanted so much for me and from me. At 24, when I decided to be a stay-at-home mom, he was disappointed. He raised me to think I could be anything, why would I make such a choice? I was the first college graduate in the family! What was I thinking?

I was thinking, I had no college debt. I had a clear identity. I was no longer lost. Until and unless something else proved worth it or we were desperate for the money, I wanted to be a full-time mom. I was making an empowered choice. I wasn't sacrificing any part of myself to be a stay-at-home mom. I wasn't leaving an exciting job or any other significant role.

Not a Permanent, Full-Time Gig

That said, I knew from the get-go that being at home full-time was a temporary gig. Kids get older; their needs change. Plus, motherhood never felt like it completely filled that inner void or fully defined my life's purpose. Parenting gave my life direction, but I still felt like something was missing. And, being home full-time with the kids could challenge my sanity like nothing I had ever previously experienced!

So, I started wondering what I could do in the meantime – just to feel mentally and emotionally stable enough to handle the roller-coaster ride of raising young children. While perusing around the bookstore (one of my favorite forms of therapy), I saw the book *Twenty-Minute Yoga Workouts* by Alice Christensen.

I hesitated. This was 1999, yoga was still pretty unusual and sometimes suspected of being a religion. But, I was compelled and made the purchase. I started reading through the book and doing the poses. From my very first triangle pose, I thought yoga was magical. I started practicing poses every single day. The effect was profound on how I felt and went about my day.

As long as I did yoga daily, I was calmer, nicer and happier. I felt like I was a better mother. I shared my enthusiasm with Dad and he said it was a fad. I was so pissed and offended and yet, suddenly very determined! I had immense pleasure in proving him completely wrong!

Nowhere Near a Fad!

After a while, when Dad understood that, indeed, it was no fad, he felt mystified and could not relate. What the hell was my fascination with yoga? We had many, many conversations about it.

I did not understand why he was so fixated on the topic and at times felt exasperated and exhausted by his questions. I thought, "What the hell does it matter? Leave me alone about it!" But, yoga had transformed my entire identity; how I breathed, walked and interacted were all influenced by my practice. Dad thought he knew me so well. He was unaccustomed and uncomfortable at being in the dark regarding such an important aspect of my life.

I now see that being pushed to have those challenging conversations made me articulate and define yoga's significance to me. It laid the groundwork for my future teaching. Having to find words, explanations that satisfied his critical mind, prepared me for my future students – who signed up willingly!

Planting More & More Seeds

Some years into my yoga practice, I became curious about Pilates. I thought I was in great shape. Pilates kicked my butt!! I could hardly do it. I wanted to be able to do it; the challenge and technique reminded me of ballet without the emotional stress of serious classes.

I started wondering what else about me was not as physically strong as I had originally thought. I investigated overall strength training. Back to the library and used bookstores! I studied and studied and loved every minute. I made notebooks, workout plans and revised continuously. I borrowed and purchased exercise videos. I found other women who were on the same path and asked for advice.

All the while, classes totally intimidated me. I was doing all these things in the privacy of my own home. I didn't want to appear foolish or wrong. I was having positive results; I did not want to feel discouraged or inept.

One day, a friend told me I should really try a class at the nearby yoga studio. She was enjoying classes and thought I would as well. I was so scared! I had been practicing yoga on my own for several years yet I still felt nervous. What if I was doing everything wrong?!

I knew it was time to take a class. There is only so much one can learn from books and videos. So, I took my self-doubt and fear with me to the yoga studio. I tried to act calm and confident. When the owner asked if I had ever taken a class, I said that I'd been practicing on my own for a while so I should be okay.

I cannot say enough that I was **SOOOO** frightened and unsure. But, I did the class. I was able to follow the instructions and keep up. Savasana (the final meditation pose) was the most difficult part because my mind was going and going. Post class – feeling brave, I bought a punch card. Within a couple months, I purchased an unlimited pass and went to class at 5:45 a.m. and then again after my husband returned home from work almost daily.

Sanity and feeling physically strong were indelibly linked. I grew more confident and self-assured. About a year into taking classes, that same friend told me I should teach yoga. I thought it was the most absurd idea I had ever heard! But, the seed had been planted. And, as luck would have it, the yoga studio was offering a teacher training. Again, with a ton of fear and uncertainty, I signed up!

Fear is my constant companion. There is nothing that I've ever pursued with absolute confidence and ease. Maybe, because fear is a constant part of me, I am used to it and don't allow it to be a permanent stop sign. Fear is annoying and scary unto itself, but it is only as powerful as I allow!

Learning How to Teach

After just a few workshops, other teachers started asking me to sub classes for them. Holy &%$!! But, I still said yes. I learned and learned from every opportunity. I had no idea why those teachers asked me or felt confident in my abilities. I had no idea if I was doing a decent job with those classes, but I was on this path and, by God, I was going for it!

My initial teacher training became a conglomeration of MANY workshops with a ton of different teachers. It took me a while to be willing to commit money and time to an actual program. The individual workshops were terrific, informative and fun. But learning from so many different perspectives also made me conscious of my deficits. I was aware of the gaps in my understanding and the effect it had on my confidence and communication with my students.

After a year of many workshops, I found that I kept returning to those offered by Kim Schwartz of The Temple of Kriya Yoga. The 12-month program entailed four, four-day trips to Chicago and tons of reading, writing, turning in tests and practicing at home. I was in heaven and so grateful for the entire family's support. Simultaneously, I also acquired a personal training certification. Income from personal training helped pay for the yoga program.

Yoga teacher training from a singular school did exactly as I had hoped. It filled in the gaps of my learning and boosted my confidence. It gave clarity and intention to my cues. I understood the bigger picture and it gave focus to my teaching style. My students responded enthusiastically and my classes grew significantly.

The Evolution Never Ceases

My personal exercise journey, teaching style and focus have all changed with time. Nothing is static. In addition to teaching yoga, I am certified and teach Pilates. Woot! Take that, Pilates! I've developed small group, women-only circuit classes that include strength training, cardio and balance. Underlying whatever I teach is a passion to continue learning and growing.

My personal path started out as a link to sanity, moved into enjoying and exploring physical challenges, and now my focus is on healthy longevity. I am excited to see what the future brings. I am excited to share the path with students who choose to join or stay with me.

You might start this path for one reason and several months or years later, your intention to continue is motivated by something else entirely. I can see how running as a kid with my dad has led to who I am today. I can see how my fear in taking classes makes me a compassionate teacher. I can see how change is valuable and necessary.

As long as we are alive, we are never done. We get to continue learning, growing, pursuing and evolving. Whether your past was pleasant or not, those experiences are a part of you. You can harness them in ways that benefit others, make you feel strong today and allow your purpose to continue to unfold.

Allow You to BE YOU in All Things

I am not the fanciest or most creative teacher. My teaching style doesn't fit into gym culture or many studios. I am not focused on getting the most intense or intricate workout. You might not even sweat in my classes.

Today, I believe form is everything. I am an alignment geek. I am driven by the idea that physical alignment leads to breathing well. As the breath travels freely through the body, stress leaves the body and mind. Booyah!

If you take my classes, you will learn intention and purpose to your movements. You will know why you are doing whatever you are doing. You will get to discern if that particular position makes sense for you in this moment – today. You will learn a lot about your anatomy. You will start to hear my voice in your head, even when you are not in my classes – in a good way. You will learn how to stand well, how to move well in your body. So that you can feel as good as possible – for as long as possible – in whatever you do.

My goal is that you will always feel physically, mentally and emotionally better post-class than you did when you first walked through the door. I hope that you will want to continue practicing yoga (or whatever form of exercise) whether it is with me, someone else or on your own.

My overall life goal is to be an excellent ambassador for healthy living. The details of what that looks like as a teacher evolve but the main goal is constant. No judgment, no comparisons and no unrealistic expectations allowed.

You are allowed to be You. You are encouraged to be You. You are celebrated for being You. And, in being a conduit for all those intentions, repeating those words aloud daily ... I remind myself to think all those same things about myself. Isn't life amazing?

XIII. MYOB: PREJUDGING, ADVISING & OVERALL "HELPFULNESS"

My body type is typically a hindrance to getting people to try my classes. Potential students take one look at me and assume there is no way I teach classes that relate to their interests, needs or abilities. They are prejudging me based on whatever stereotype or past experience in their life.

It's okay, I get it. I make my pitch anyway. I relay that I am very adept at teaching the beginner. If they have been moderately active, then my classes are totally doable. I let them know that my typical student is a positive example of healthy aging; a polite way of saying they are older than me.

My average yoga student is between 50 and 75. Often, they have been active but never done yoga. They have been walking, golfing, skiing or biking and are curious about yoga. A doctor, friend or some random person has recommended it. They have arthritis, knee and/or hip replacements, fibromyalgia or plantar fasciitis. They are cancer or heart attack survivors. They come from all walks of life, careers and life experiences.

I am honored that they trust me to guide their bodies through movement. They are doing what I ask of them with a willingness to explore, to test the waters. Sometimes, I ask them to visit a move they haven't done in decades or ever in their lifetime, yet they give it a go. Sometimes, the attempt results in the class erupting in laughter but it is all good.

We test incrementally. I was never a diver. I don't just jump into the pool – it's not my style. I ease my way in – allowing my body to adjust and see if it can handle the temperature. I apply the same methods to yoga, Pilates and strength training. This process allows the body a chance to assess, organize and participate safely.

A Model Shift

The photos on my website used to only be of me in poses. But, that was not a selling point. I teach basic yoga and Pilates in a community center. We will most likely never put our foot behind our head, do a handstand or a full forearm balance while in class. If nothing else, there is not enough blank wall space!

Now my website also has photos of my students. I tell all my potentials to take a look. Real people, not size zero, fitness magazine models take my classes. Although, I think my students should be on the cover of every fitness magazine. They are also definitions of health and fitness! But, our world can be ridiculous in its limited definition of healthy.

Exercising and feeling healthy is attainable ... period. No one has to be stick thin to qualify as healthy or take an exercise class. Grrrr!

So, as you peruse classes, teachers and fellow peers, please don't prejudge based on size in either direction. Our size does not tell the entire story of our health. Are we able to move well? Do we have the desire, energy and stamina to move? Do we feel reasonably agile and moderately balanced? Do we feel enthusiastic about our life? These are some of the qualities to look for and that define good health.

Being "Helpful"

In my grandparents' world, anyone bigger than them was overweight. They could be funny except they also judged anyone bigger than themselves, especially if said person was younger. Why couldn't so and so control their appetites? It was bizarre and sad to me.

I remember being told a story that Zady once promised Bubbe a fur coat if she lost a certain amount of weight. She lost the weight, got the fur and quickly put all the weight back on – *not helpful*.

Today, I wonder: why did Zady think he had any business giving Bubbe that kind of goal? I guess she told him that exactly – and still got the fur!

Right after my 40th birthday, a male student (whom I adore) happened to be curious, and asked me about the sudden extra bit around my middle. I felt devastated. Because, of course, I had noticed a little something right there. I was trying to understand it myself. How and why did it all of a sudden appear? I am not sure if he felt it was okay to ask because I am slender. Let me say this simply: it is never okay. Let me repeat: IT IS NEVER OKAY!!

MYOB: Mind Your Own Business

On your path to health and wellness, you might feel inspired to motivate others to join you. Enthusiasm is contagious; you don't need to say one single word. Being helpful is responding to people's questions and no more. Not one of us knows the secret formula to help someone else on their path.

Be available. Be positive. Be encouraging. Don't provide goals that they never asked for. Don't notice aloud their weight gain. Trust me – they know.

They are looking for an incentive and are seeking your help? Beautiful. Ask them what kinds of things motivate them. Help them brainstorm but don't create specific goals for them.

Aside from the previously stated reasons in the "Strategies" chapter, I am the first in line for food at a party and first to rest if I am tired in an exercise class. I have nothing to prove and want to model that there is no shame in eating or resting. My behavior gives others permission to do so. My joy in eating healthy and exercising will be motivating – or not, but I am not here to preach to or judge anyone.

I am stubborn. No one can convince me to do anything long term that I don't personally buy into. No one can be convinced into changing their lifestyle unless they know it and decide it for themselves. So, be a positive example. Be happy. Love others as they are – today and…

MYOB!

XIV. WITNESSING TRANSFORMATION: MY AMAZING STUDENTS

The most amazing and inspiring aspect of my job is having the constant opportunity to witness positive transformation amongst my students. They transform in attitude, strength, endurance, knowledge and energy level. It doesn't matter that I'm completely biased – I know they are incredible! I would have loved to include all couple hundred of them in this book but knowing that would be impossible, I asked eight!

I chose women who I knew represented the group as a whole. Barb, Lauren, Julie, Kendi, Anne, Mahshid, Mackenzie and Jan are every woman. They come from all walks of life and backgrounds. They vary in struggles and strengths. What binds them together is their role modeling of positivity and commitment to living healthy – in a way they define. I hope you see yourself in their stories. I hope you find inspiration in their stories – as I have. I wanted to share a little extra about each one of them from my perspective.

Barbara and Lauren Cason were among my very first students at the community center. For years, I looked at them in awe that they continued to sign up for my classes. Their abilities have always exceeded the scope of what I teach. Yet, they continue to sign up. It still amazes me. I love to tease Lauren in front of the other students because she is so bendy. I love to brag that Barb is 60 and among the strongest in the group of circuit ladies! I have only known them together. They come as a pair, working out side by side for years. Their relationship is beautiful and inspiring.

Julie Chesis is the wonderful woman who got me back to personal training and was the inspiration for me to teach small group, women-only circuit classes. Julie adds humor and fun to any group. Her energy is completely contagious. Julie shifted from only feeling comfortable with one-on-one workouts to requiring the company of the other women. The mere **idea** of working out alone with me inspires her to turn around and threaten to return home! I had no real understanding how scary the entire process has been for her until reading her story for this book. Julie's commitment to exercise and healthier living is impressive and motivating. Her inner transformation is phenomenal and inspiring!

Kendria Elliott is a wonder to me. I whine when I get a cold. No matter Kendi's physical health or other hurdles that life's thrown at her, she is strong, positive and humble. I feel as though I've witnessed Kendi in so many physical phases but her essence, her strength and faith are always there and seem to only grow stronger. No matter the obstacle, she keeps returning to class and making it work. Kendi is an unwavering role model to all who surround her.

Anne Schultz shocked the hell out of me when she told me her age! Then, I proceeded to see the exact same reaction reflected in all of the other circuit ladies' expressions! Anne typically lifts more weight and has more endurance than all of us! Anne has worked with such focus and determination at honing her alignment. She is a prime example that it is never too late to learn a new way of doing something. Anne came to me strong but now she stands taller. Any threat of a dowager's hump has been eliminated. Booyah! I want to be Anne when I grow up!

Mahshid Hesani came to me tired and down. She knew that she needed to make changes in her life but had no idea of where to start. Mahshid had so many questions and was like a sponge with the information. She took to yoga, Pilates, strength training with a vengeance and became alive before my eyes. I can hardly visualize the "before Mahshid" because today she is vibrant, positive and strong. It's like a light bulb went off and only continues to grow brighter. To say that Mahshid is enthusiastic is an understatement!

Raising a daughter in today's society when your business is fitness is one scary endeavor and yet, **Mackenzie** handles herself with grace and poise. She is everything I wish I could have been at her age. I am so proud of her and look forward to watching her grow into the wonderful adult I know she is becoming.

Jan Harness and I knew one another as fellow congregants at our local synagogue. Once a year, Jan attended my yoga class offered at our synagogue's women's retreat. And then one day, Jan signed up for my women-only circuit classes. During her first class, I knew she was really tempted to leave midway through – that's probably putting it lightly! I just silently prayed that she would see it through and quietly encouraged her. She made it through and thankfully continued!

I watched a woman transform before my eyes. A begrudging exerciser became a woman who attended class at every opportunity. With time, Jan added yoga, Pilates and mindful eating to her healthy living routine. I saw a woman grow more comfortable in fitted clothing. I watched her enjoy the sight of her changing body. Jan grew stronger and more confident on all levels.

Then one day after circuit class Jan told me, "Sweetie, you need to write a book." People/students have been telling me that I needed to write a book almost from the beginning of my teaching career. I have always taken it as a compliment but never as a serious pursuit. I responded, "I have no idea what I could possibly write about." Jan responded, "Get a piece of paper and pen. I'll tell you **exactly** what you need to write about." And, she did. ☺

This book was birthed because of Jan's constant cheering, advising, idea giving, editing, interviewing and so much more. I am so grateful to have Jan by my side. I hope to spend many more years together, pursuing healthy longevity and sharing our positive vision with others.

XV. NOW, BE ON YOUR WAY!

Now is your time to shine.

I hope you feel empowered.
I hope you feel strong.
I hope you feel compassionate toward yourself.
I hope you know more about yourself now than you did before.
I hope you continue to learn more about yourself.
I hope you share the best of who you are with others.

You are enough. You are wonderful.
Keep striving.
Keep trying.
You are worthy of the effort.
You are worthy of the investment of time, money and energy.
You are worthy.
You can do anything that you truly want and are willing to do.

I hope you believe in yourself.
I hope you surprise yourself.
I hope that someday I get to meet you.

With Much Gratitude and Many Hugs,
Shanna

XVI. RESOURCES

Included:

My Daily Food Routine

Homework: Creating an Ever-Changing Health Map

Incomplete List of Truths in Almost Every Yoga Pose

Incomplete List of "Safe" Gorging Ideas!

Contact Shanna

Other Helpful Websites

My Daily Food Routine ... as of this moment

I want to preface this by saying I think my eating habits are outside of the norm! I have no expectation that most people will like the taste or texture of my smoothie concoction or want a ton of fruit in their salad. Please don't feel limited. As stated earlier, this is how I enjoy eating. I love having a predictable routine. As I learn new information, I tweak, no big overhaul – ever. There are many, many paths to living healthy.

I enjoy having a predictable routine of fairly clean eating. As mentioned previously, I really notice what happens to my body and mind if I go "off the map." One day recently, I drank two cups of dark roast, bold flavor caffeinated coffee (which I never do). We purchased a Keurig® and I was excited about using it.

The after effect was awful. I was tired and wired simultaneously. I had the inner shakes and tremors. It took a great deal of awareness to keep my energy focused and grounded rather than all over the place. My body had no experience in processing that much caffeine so it felt abused. And, I still had to teach yoga! Needless to say, my limit was immediately adjusted to one cup if any! I've expanded my Keurig use for tea and making oatmeal!

I have no goal to acclimate my body to high doses of caffeine but it is another example of the importance of tweaking, regardless of the direction! Your body is used to the status quo so don't shock it … inspire it!

Food is also one of my family's primary expenses – so a lot of the ingredients are on the expensive side. However, I know some are curious so here goes!

No recipe is static. For the smoothie, I have changed the fruit and type of protein powder over the years. Seeds and greens are a newer addition. Cinnamon and clove are included for potential anti-inflammatory properties.

6:20 a.m. - BREAKFAST - Smoothie Recipe:

- ¼ cup coconut water
- ¼ cup pomegranate, acai or aloe juice
- 1¼ cups water
- 1 T each hemp, ground chia and ground flax seeds
- 2 T plant-based protein powder
- 1 t cocoa
- ¼ to ½ t cinnamon
- ¼ t clove
- 1 t Stevia

- ½ banana
- ¼ cup each frozen blueberries, cherries, mango and pineapple
- Handful of washed greens
- 1 T all-natural peanut butter

To save time:

I make one month's worth of individual cups of:

- 2 T protein powder
- 1 t cocoa
- ½ t cinnamon
- ¼ t clove
- 1 t Stevia

I make one month's worth of individual freezer bags of:
¼ cup each frozen blueberries, cherries, mango and pineapple

Daily process:

Every morning around 6:15 a.m., I (or my wonderful husband) put the liquids into the blender, add the seeds, add contents of the powder cup, ½ banana, fruit, washed greens and peanut butter. Blend and blend, pour and drink! I love using a straw.

SNACK (maybe)

IF I need a mid-morning snack between teaching two classes back to back:

Spoonful of peanut butter with honey or a Zing® bar: **www.zingbars.com.**

When it comes to bars (and many packaged meals), I look at net carbs, which I define as total carbohydrates minus protein and fiber. So, the Zing bars are around 10 net carbs. I wouldn't want any bar that had more than 15 net carbs.

The Zing bars are easy for me to digest between teaching classes without feeling heavy in my belly or creating that high/low impact on my blood sugar. They have a handful of flavors that don't contain dairy (for those who prefer or have an intolerance). I enjoy the dark chocolate hazelnut and coconut cashew crisp flavors most.

PRE-WORKOUT (maybe)

Before attending a class and after teaching one or two classes, I might consume Vega® Sport Pre-Workout Energizer Powder found at **www.vegasport.com** and possibly a small spoonful of peanut butter with honey. This all depends on my energy level and anticipated intensity of the upcoming class.

Noon or 2 p.m. LUNCH

Post teaching morning class(es) and working out, either around noon or 2 p.m. depending on my schedule, it's *Big Salad Time*! These ingredients also change greatly with the seasons. Every Monday, Wednesday and Friday I make two days' worth of salads in reusable plastic containers. The ingredients go into each bowl as I chop and separate. On Sundays, I make a single salad, improvise or eat something like a Subway® sandwich or Panera Bread® salad.

Big Salad "Recipe"

Per bowl, a handful of:

- Washed greens
- Chopped celery,
- ½ cucumber
- Sliced carrots
- Handful of cherry tomatoes
- Chopped strawberries, possibly grapes
- Mango, pineapple or ½ an apple (depending on how much other fruit is in it)
- ½ an avocado
- Lean protein such as tuna, salmon or low-sodium deli meat
- Seasoned with balsamic vinegar and sometimes other spices

3:30 p.m. SNACK

Depending on what time I ate my salad and how active my day has been, I might need a small meal prior to teaching my evening class(es). It could be one of the following:

- 1 bowl of Skinny Pop® popcorn (**www.skinnypop.com**) with or without butter-flavored olive oil – my favorite is from our local Olive Tree store: **www.olivetreekc.com**
- A Zing bar (if I haven't had one earlier in the day) **www.zingbars.com**
- A couple of eggs in whatever variety, i.e. boiled, scrambled
- 1 chia seed waffle with peanut butter and strawberry preserves
- An apple with peanut butter

- Small bowl of oatmeal. I am currently enjoying Hot & Fit Cereal™ Earnest Eats® blends – **www.earnesteats.com**. I typically add a small spoonful of peanut butter and strawberry preserves
- ¼ cup of pumpkin seeds
- Justin's® single serving pack of peanut or almond butter **www.justins.com**

7:30 p.m. DINNER

After teaching my evening classes on Monday through Thursday, we try to keep things simple and easy. Examples are one of the following options:

- Prepackaged frozen chicken patty or grilled chicken breast, ½ steam bag of veggies, ½ Garden Lites™ butternut squash soufflé. We find the soufflés in the frozen food section at our local Whole Foods Market®. Check out **www.gardenlite.com** for other varieties
- Grilled fish, ½ steam bag of veggies, quinoa
- Eggs and ½ steam bag of veggies

Criteria I look for in DINNER convenience foods:

- No dairy (due to intolerance)
- Not heavy with garlic or onion (they also irritate my system)
- Sodium – around 500 mg or less
- Protein – around 20 grams
- Fiber – at least 5 grams
- Fat – I'm not terribly concerned with this. I keep the ingredients in mind. If nuts or olive oil are in the recipe, then fat content will be on the higher side. If I can't find a

good reason for the quantity of fat, then I don't purchase the item.

Favorite Desserts (the key is to stick to the serving size):

- Garden Lites' veggie muffins - zucchini chocolate flavor: **www.gardenlites.com**. I add strawberries or strawberry preserves
- Miss J's™ Truffley treats: **www.ohyesyoucandy.com**
- Trader Joe's® sea salt and turbinado sugar dark chocolate covered almonds: **www.traderjoes.com**
- Hail Merry® Tarte – **www.hailmerry.com**

Please let me know your quick, easy, and healthy tips!

Homework: Creating an Ever-Changing Health Map

As you go through the process of creating a health map, please remember that it is not static. Your life is constantly changing and your priorities are allowed to change along the way. Writing out your typical day for several days gives you an idea of what your life looks like today. You'll want to keep it as basic as possible. Don't count out calories. Just keep track of perceived quantities and characteristics of each meal. The intention of this exercise is to grow awareness, observe patterns and identify what matters most to you. This is not an exercise in judgment. You are not bad! Remember, you are a *practicer*.

Include the following information:

1. Amount and quality of sleep (include how many times you woke up)
2. Wake-up time and mood
3. Level of appetite on a scale of one to 10. One being you couldn't care less about food and 10 being famished! Write down the time of your meal with type and general quantities
4. General activities/tasks/duties that fill the time between meals and overall energy level
5. Repeat numbers three and four until the end of the day
6. Bed time

After completing the above exercise, take a look at it. Notice your feelings around reading through it. Ponder the questions below. There is no need to go through the questions all at once. Visit them as you feel ready.

Sleep

- Do you have a regular/predictable sleep schedule and wake-up time?
- How would you describe the quality of your sleep?
- Is there anything you would like to do differently around your sleep schedule or quality of sleep?
- What do you think of as positive sleep habits and could you easily incorporate them?
- How realistic would it be to go to sleep and wake up around the same time each day? Does that idea even sound appealing?
- Do the timing of your last meal prior to bed and types of foods consumed affect the quality of your sleep?

Food

- What foods do you think were consumed out of habit and what foods were fully enjoyed?
- Were the enjoyable foods truly pleasurable or a trigger for gorging?
- What foods are absolute keepers? You can't envision an enjoyable life without those particular foods. Do not allow guilt to enter. Keep those special foods in your life!
- What foods did you eat out of convenience? Are you interested in replacing them with healthier options?
- What foods would you define as healthier options? Would you call them pleasant, tasty and affordable as well as healthy?
- How would you easily incorporate the habit of purchasing, preparing and eating those healthier options?

- Do you eat your meals around the same times each day? Is the idea appealing and easily doable?
- Do you crave variety? Or, are you comfortable with routine?
- Would you like to go to the grocery store as a *field trip*? This is an opportunity to explore items that look appealing and allows time to read labels. The visit can be an individual exercise or one done as a family.

Energy Level

- Do you feel that you have the energy to regularly accomplish all that matters most to you?
- If you had the energy to accomplish all that mattered most to you, how would your life be different?
- If you have a typical energy dip, when is it? What food/activity preceded it? What did you do about it – how did you deal with or manage it?

Activities/Duties

- What activities or tasks fill your day?
- Do you find the majority of your day pleasant?
- Do you feel "in-charge" regarding the flow of your day and the activities that fill it?
- Are there realistic ways to make your day even more enjoyable and less stressful?
- Do you have a support network?
- Can any of your duties shift to a team effort rather than solely done by you?
- Are there gaps available for self-defined enjoyable exercise?

- Are there any typical tasks that are time-fillers and energy stealers but are not completely necessary to focus on? Sometimes we create more "have to's" than exist in reality.
- Do you have "me-time" every day? If yes, is there a noticeable, positive impact on your life as well as for those your life affects? If no, why not and do you see value in creating it?
- What would you most like to tweak about your day? How would that make your day and life better?

Motivation for Change

- What is the first thing in your typical day that would be almost effortless to tweak?
- How would the tweak improve your life? What is your buy-in?
- What interests you most? Prioritize the following:
  - A reduced number on the scale
  - A smaller clothing size
  - Increased energy level
  - Enhanced mood
  - Your choice _____
- How would your life improve today if you accomplished your top selected goal?
- When was the last time in your life that you lived in that state of being?
- If you ever lived for a significant time in that state of being does your memory of it match up with your hopes if it occurred today?
- How is your life different today?
- What do you think are the major roadblocks that have prevented you from living the life you want?

- How will you manage those roadblocks differently from this day forward?

Successful, positive and lasting change occurs a little at a time. Make sure that you can define its worth to you and that your impetus is positive!

Incomplete List of Truths in Almost Every Yoga Pose

In my yoga teacher training, Tadasana or *Mountain pose* was taught as the model for every other pose. Another way of understanding Mountain pose is viewing it as standing tall. Learning how to consistently stand tall (as well as sit tall) with awareness can assist and minimize the common aches and pains easily acquired in everyday life.

Some tips to assist with and quiet those frequent aches and pains:

- In a standing position, align your feet so that your toes are mostly pointing forward or you are slightly pigeon-toed. The *center line* of each foot points forward and those two lines are parallel with one another.
- Soften your knees and shift your body weight into your heels.
- Lift your toes and press the inner lines of your feet downward with the intention of bringing energy up your legs. This will inspire the inner line of your legs to engage (think inner thighs).
- Add on pressing the outer edges of your feet downward. This will inspire the outer lines of your legs to engage.
- Add on pressing across the width of each heel. This should cause the base of the glutes to engage – lengthening the back spine and releasing the sacrum downward (a triangular bone at your lower back). You might feel a release of tension if your lower back tends to tense.
- Add on pressing across the ball mounds of your toes. This should engage the pelvic floor and lengthen the front spine.

- All these actions should cause muscular energy in your legs to ascend. You are drawing energy and power up from the ground and your body should grow in length and inner space.
- Aligning the joints: drawing energy up engages the quadriceps (front thigh muscle) upwards which should correct any subtle misalignment between the hip, knee and ankle in each leg.
- These actions combined lighten the load carried by all the joints and clear the channels for energy to travel.
- If you are hypermobile in the joints, then be extra aware of hyperextension. This especially occurs in knees and elbows – you might feel a bulge behind the knees or inner elbows. You want to be careful to not "lock" the joints, as this also creates tension.
- Draw your inner shoulder blades toward one another. This will send your shoulders back and lift the sternum forward and upward.
- Engage muscles below the armpits (the serratus anterior) whenever bearing weight. This will connect muscles of the front body to the back body, inspire abdominal muscles to engage as well as remove load from smaller muscles around your neck.
  - o The idea is to draw the shoulders down by using muscles below the shoulders versus sending the shoulders down via muscles from above.

All the actions above should result in the center of the ears lining up over the center of the shoulders, which line up over the hips, which line up over the heels. Voila! Welcome to Mountain pose! I still think of Mountain pose as one of my most personally challenging poses to consistently do well.

Once students are aligned, I give the following three cues no matter the position:

1) Ascend energy from the ground up (the spine elongates)
2) Direct peripheral energy in toward the midline of your body (the spine elongates even more)
3) Radiate energy from your midline to your periphery (this balances the power and openness in the position)

The cues above are not a cure for anything; they are a management style. We can take the Mountain pose stance and apply it to lunges, push-ups, Warrior II, putting away groceries and driving our car! Living more physically aware improves the quality of our life. Moving with proper alignment lessens aches and pains. Excellent posture helps us breathe better, which alone decreases our stress level. Many students tell me that they measure taller at the doctor's office merely by standing with proper alignment!

Say no to hunching! Give the above cues a whirl. Look at yourself on profile to a mirror and position your posture with a straight line from the center of your ear over your shoulder over your hip over your heel.

Now, place a hard-cover book on your head and walk around! Stop walking, sit down and stand up without the book dropping. I dare you! Next step: find a good yoga class!

Incomplete List of "Safe" Gorging Ideas!

Anything can be done too much. Some things are just less punishing! I love to feast, to delve into subjects, to immerse my brain and senses. So I am always on the lookout for activities to partake with no regret! I look for things that feel enriching on all levels. Below are some expanded ideas from the Strategies chapter. Please add and share ideas of your own!

Visit libraries. Gather a stack of books on whatever topic. Find a comfy chair and get cozy. Feast! Look through the music. Check out the art on the walls and shelves. Take a look at the book lists and staff favorites. I love perusing the staff reads!

Park or museum hop! Check out all of the parks and museums in your area. Track your visits as accomplishments! It will make you an incredible resource of information for your friends. Research and create a wish list of local places you have yet to visit. Make each visit an adventure! I turned museum visits into scavenger hunts. Prior to looking around, we always visited the museum shop. I let each kid pick out five postcards of works they found compelling. Then, we proceeded to hunt for those 10 items! Meanwhile, I got the chance to revel in the art! The kids still remember those visits as fun.

Bookstores! I have always found bookstores comforting and today they are even better. Aside from containing books on every imaginable topic and a variety of music and movies, there are games! I find a great deal of inspiration for family-fun inspecting all the games. It will also leave you prepared to host a game night with your friends!

Walk outside whenever possible! Discover your neighborhood and your neighbors. I am pretty sure that some in my neighborhood only know me as the "walking lady." Recently, I attended a high school football game and the ticket sales lady commented that I looked so familiar. As a line of people waited behind me, she realized that she had seen me walk by her house many days!

Free concerts! Summer is a fabulous time for this. We have them offered in parks almost every weekend during the summer.

Window shop ... after hours! You won't be able to spend any money. Yet, you'll get exercise and return home feeling inspired with ideas.

Check out free or inexpensive community classes! Community colleges and centers are great for this but so are home improvement stores, libraries, craft stores, etc.

I really love looking around on **www.Etsy.com**. All that creativity in one place! It is so impressive and expands my mind.

Do any of these ideas resonate with you? What else would you add to this list? Send me your ideas!

Contact Shanna

I would love to speak at your event! Please contact me for:

Speaking engagements, fitness/health workshops and symposiums, Skype into book group discussions and the like!

Press kits and media relations: jan@healthyheartandmind.com

Website: www.HealthyHeartAndMind.com

Blog: http://healthyheartandmind.wordpress.com

Email: shanna@healthyheartandmind.com

Twitter: @ShannaHaun

Other Helpful Websites:

Teacher training: Temple of Kriya Yoga teacher training: http://yogakriya.org/php/hytths.php

Favorite athletic clothing: Lululemon Athletica®: http://shop.lululemon.com/home.jsp

For yoga props: YogaAccessories.com®: http://www.yogaaccessories.com

ABOUT THE AUTHOR

Shanna Haun, RYT, is a registered yoga teacher with a certification from Temple of Kriya Yoga in Chicago. She has been teaching yoga and fitness classes since 2005 with an emphasis on making them approachable and accessible to students of all levels. Shanna's popular presentations include morning warm-up sessions, keynotes and workshops. She presents the way she teaches – engaging the audience with activities matched to their needs, weaving yoga and gentle stretches into her presentations.

Shanna is a native of Overland Park, Kan., and gives back to her community as an active volunteer. She received a B.A. in Psychology from the University of Kansas.

Shanna is married to an incredible partner, Matt Haun, and together they have two terrific kids, Mackenzie and Aaron, and an attention-seeking dog, Bailey!

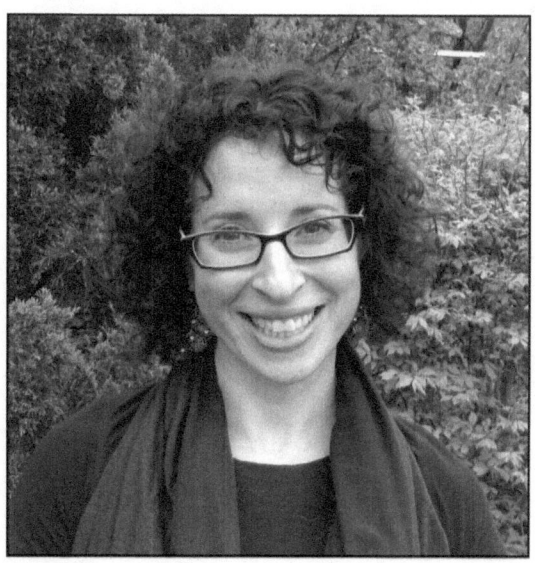